Neural Cell Culture

The Practical Approach Series

SERIES EDITORS

D. RICKWOOD
Department of Biology, University of Essex
Wivenhoe Park, Colchester, Essex CO4 3SQ, UK

B. D. HAMES
Department of Biochemistry and Molecular Biology
University of Leeds, Leeds LS2 9JT, UK

★ **indicates new and forthcoming titles**

Affinity Chromatography
Anaerobic Microbiology
Animal Cell Culture
  (2nd Edition)
Animal Virus Pathogenesis
Antibodies I and II
★ Basic Cell Culture
Behavioural Neuroscience
Biochemical Toxicology
★ Bioenergetics
Biological Data Analysis
Biological Membranes
Biomechanics — Materials
Biomechanics — Structures
  and Systems
Biosensors
★ Carbohydrate Analysis
  (2nd Edition)
Cell–Cell Interactions
★ The Cell Cycle
★ Cell Growth and Apoptosis
Cellular Calcium

Cellular Interactions in
  Development
Cellular Neurobiology
Clinical Immunology
Crystallization of Nucleic Acids
  and Proteins
★ Cytokines (2nd Edition)
The Cytoskeleton
Diagnostic Molecular Pathology
  I and II
Directed Mutagenesis
★ DNA Cloning 1: Core Techniques
  (2nd Edition)
★ DNA Cloning 2: Expression
  Systems (2nd Edition)
★ DNA Cloning 3: Complex
  Genomes (2nd Edition)
★ DNA Cloning 4: Mammalian
  Systems (2nd Edition)
Electron Microscopy in Biology
Electron Microscopy in
  Molecular Biology
Electrophysiology

Neural Cell Culture
A Practical Approach

Edited by

JAMES COHEN

Division of Anatomy and Cell Biology,
UMDS – Guy's Campus, London Bridge, London SE1 9RT

and

GRAHAM P. WILKIN

Department of Biochemistry,
Imperial College of Science, Technology and Medicine,
Kensington, London SW7 2AZ

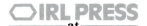
OXFORD UNIVERSITY PRESS
Oxford New York Tokyo

Oxford University Press, Walton Street, Oxford OX2 6DP

Oxford   New York
Athens   Auckland   Bangkok   Bombay
Calcutta   Cape Town   Dar es Salaam   Delhi
Florence   Hong Kong   Istanbul   Karachi
Kuala Lumpur   Madras   Madrid   Melbourne
Mexico City   Nairobi   Paris   Singapore
Taipei   Tokyo   Toronto
and associated companies in
Berlin   Ibadan

Oxford is a trade mark of Oxford University Press

Published in the United States
by Oxford University Press Inc., New York

A catalogue record for this book is available from the British Library

Library of Congress Cataloging-in-Publication Data
Neural cell culture: a practical approach/edited by James Cohen and
Graham P. Wilkin.
(Practical approach series; 163)
Includes bibliographical references and index.
1. Neurons—Growth—Laboratory manuals.   2. Cell culture—
Laboratory manuals.   I. Cohen, James, Dr.   II. Wilkin, Graham P.
III. Series.
[DNLM: 1. Neurons—cytology.   2. Tissue Culture—methods.
WL 102.5 N4922   1995]
QP357.N47   1995   612.8'0724—dc20   95-39515
ISBN 0 19 963485 8 (Hbk)
ISBN 0 19 963484 x (Pbk)

Typeset by Footnote Graphics, Warminster, Wilts
Printed in Great Britain by Information Press Ltd, Eynsham, Oxon.

Preface

Faced with the immense complexity and cellular heterogeneity of the vertebrate nervous system, tissue culture model systems have long been sought with which to study the properties of the many varieties of neural cell types. In fact, tissue culture was pioneered as a research technique almost a century ago, by the US biologist Ross Harrison, in a classic study which helped resolve a controversy in neurobiology. The widespread adoption of *in vitro* techniques by neurobiologists had to wait another 70 years or so, before the advantages could be fully exploited. This depended to a great extent on technical developments; of reliable CO_2-gassed tissue culture incubators, defined media, and inexpensive, disposable cultureware, that improved cell viability, sterility, and reproducibility. Moreover, because the growth and differentiation of most neural cell types is anchorage-dependent, it also greatly benefited, over the last 15 years, from the identification and purification of natural adhesive molecules, including components of the extracellular matrix. In addition, over the same period, the increasing availability of antibodies that enable the phenotype of isolated neural cells to be unambiguously identified and, in some instances, separated into pure populations, has enormously increased the power of cell culture as a research technique. Finally, the recent explosion of information on the specific growth factor requirements of distinct subpopulations of neural cells, both neurons and glia, and the availabilty of recombinant factors, has enabled culture media to be supplemented to enhance the survival and growth of many cell cultures previously perceived as difficult or impossible to maintain *in vitro*. As a result of these developments, today, the use of neural cell cultures impinges on almost every aspect of neurobiological research and is increasingly becoming an essential experimental tool in helping unravel the underlying mechanisms of fundamental processes governing the development and function of both the normal and damaged nervous system. Also there is a growing awareness of the need for more appropriate culture model systems derived from distinct regions of the nervous system that take account of its functional and cellular heterogeneity.

A manual such as this one can be one of two things: either an exhaustive but necessarily superficial survey of all currently available methods for culturing neural cells, or a selective but thorough guide to the culture of particular populations of cells that are representative of the nervous system's diversity. We have opted for the latter, and in particular focused on classes of cells, both neurons and glia, that have recently been the focus of much interest in studies of nervous system function in health and disease. This has enabled us to include methods covering a wide diversity of neural tissues, with the objective of making a similarly diverse range of techniques available. It is our

9. Microglia: the tissue macrophage of the CNS   107
M. Nicola Woodroofe and M. Louise Cuzner

10. Brain endothelium   121
David Male

Contents

16. Schwann cell culture

Louise Morgan

Contributors

ROGER BARKER
Department of Neurology, Addenbrooke's Hospital, Hills Road, Cambridge CB2 2QQ, UK.

EVELYNE BLOCH-GALLEGO
INSERM U.382, IBDM, Campus de Luminy–CASE907, 13288 Marseille Cedex 09, France.

ANNE L. CALOF
Department of Anatomy and Neurobiology and Developmental Biology Centre, University of California College of Medicine, Irvine, CA 92717-1275, USA.

WILLIAM CAMU
Biochimie CNRS, INSERM, BP 5051, 34033 Montpellier Cedex, France.

MARTIN A. CAMBRAY-DEAKIN
Department of Biomedical Science, University of Sheffield, Sheffield S10 2TN, UK.

SUSANA COHEN-CORY
Mental Retardation Research Centre, 760 Westwood Plaza, University of California, Los Angeles, California 90024.

ELLEN J. COLLARINI
MRC Laboratory for Molecular Cell Biology, University College London, Gower Street, London WC1E 6BT, UK.

M. LOUISE CUZNER
Department of Neurochemistry, Institute of Neurology, 1 Wakefield Street, London WC1N 1RJ, UK.

ALUN. M. DAVIES
School of Biological and Medical Sciences, University of St Andrews, St Andrews KY16 9TS, UK.

MURIEL DELANNET
Institut Jacques Monod, Université Paris 7, Tour 43, 2 Place Jussieu, 75251 Paris, France.

JEAN-LOUP DUBAND
Institut Jacques Monod, Université Paris 7, Tour 43, 2 Place Jussieu, 75251 Paris, France.

MELINDA K. GORDON
Department of Biology, 138, Biology Building, University of Iowa, Iowa City, Iowa 52242, USA.

Contributors

JOSE L. GUEVARA
Department of Biology, 138, Biology Building, University of Iowa, Iowa City, Iowa 52242, USA.

CHRISTOPHER E. HENDERSON
INSERM U.382, IBDM, Campus de Luminy–CASE907, 13288 Marseille Cedex 09, France.

WARREN D. HIRST
Department of Biochemistry, Imperial College of Science, Technology and Medicine, Kensington, London SW7 2AZ, UK.

ALAN JOHNSON
Department of Anatomy, University of Cambridge, Cambridge, CB2 3DY, UK.

LAURA LILLIEN
Medical College of Pennsylvania, Department of Anatomy, 3200 Henry Avenue, Philadelphia PA 19129, USA.

M. CECILIA LJUNGBERG
Department of Biochemistry, Imperial College of Science, Technology and Medicine, Kensington, London SW7 2AZ, UK.

DAVID MALE
Department of Neuropathology, Institute of Psychiatry, De Crespigny Park, Denmark Hill, London SE5 8AF, UK.

DEREK R. MARRIOTT
Department of Biochemistry, Imperial College of Science, Technology and Medicine, Kensington, London SW7 2AZ, UK.

FREDERIQUE MONIER
Institut Jacques Monod, Université Paris 7, Tour 43, 2 Place Jussieu, 75251 Paris, France.

LOUISE MORGAN
Esai London Laboratories, Bernard Katz Building, University College London, Gower Street, London WC1E 6BT, UK.

RAE NISHI
Department of Cell and Developmental Biology, Oregon Health Sciences University, 3181 SW Sam Jackson Park Road, Portland, OR 97201, USA.

M. JILL SAFFREY
Department of Biology, The Open University, Milton Keynes MK7 6AA, UK.

CLIVE SVENDSEN
MRC Cambridge Centre for Brain Repair, The Adrian Bldg., Robinson Way, Cambridge CB2 2PY, UK.

M. NICOLA WOODROOFE
Division of Biomedical Sciences, Sheffield Hallam University, Sheffield S1 1WB, UK.

Abbreviations

AraC	cytosine arabinoside
BBSS	bicarbonate-buffered salt solution
BME	basal medium with Earle's salts
BSA	bovine serum albumin
BSS	balanced salts solution
CM	culture medium
CMF–HBSS	calcium- and magnesium-free Hank's balanced salt solution
CMF–PBS	calcium- and magnesium-free phosphate-buffered saline
CNTF	ciliary neurotrophic factor
CSF	colony stimulating factor
DAB	3′3 diaminobenzidine HCl
DMEM(−CM)	Dulbecco's modified Eagles medium (calcium-, magnesium-free)
EBS(S)	Earle's balanced salts (solution)
EGF	epidermal growth factor
EtOH	ethanol
FCS	fetal calf serum
(b)FGF	(basic) fibroblast growth factor
GAD	glutamic acid decarboxylase
GalC	galactocerebroside
GAP-43	growth-associated protein 43
GFAP	glial fibrillary acidic protein
GPA	growth promoting activity
HBSS	Hank's balanced salt solution
HC	Huntingdon's Chorea
IN	inner nuclear layer (of retina)
IPNs	immediate neuronal precursors
LPS	lipopolysaccharide
MEM	Eagle's minimal essential medium
NGF	nerve growth factor
NGS	normal goat serum
NS	nasal septum
NSE	non-specific esterase
OE	olfactory epithelium
ONL	outer nuclear layer (of retina)
ORNs	olfactory receptor neurons
OT	olfactory turbinates

Abbreviations

PBS	phosphate-buffered saline
PD	Parkinson's disease
PDGF (AA)	platelet-derived growth factor (AA homodimer)
TLCK	tosyl lysyl cholecystokinin
VM	ventral mesencephalon

I. CNS neurons

Cerebellar Granule cells

MARTIN A. CAMBRAY-DEAKIN

1. Introduction

From a casual scan of the literature, it appears that rodent cerebellar granule cell cultures are being used in increasing numbers to address different questions in neurobiology. There are good reasons for this: the cultures are relatively easy to prepare, the starting material is neonatal rat pup thus avoiding the use of pregnant females to provide embryos, the resulting cultures are almost entirely of one cell type, and the cells produced are of relatively high yield for a neuronal culture. Granule cell cultures clearly constitute an excellent model system for studies of structural, biochemical, and electrophysiological development (1,2). In some cases the highly ordered structure of the cerebellum allows parallel studies to be performed *in vivo* or in slice preparations.

2. Initial preparation

2.1 Stock solutions

The routine of cell culture is greatly facilitated by the preparation of stock solutions of buffer and media components. We find that all our stock solutions can be prepared non-aseptically and stored at $-20\,^{\circ}C$ in aliquots for at least two to three months without noticeable problems. With the exception of poly-D-lysine all of the components are diluted where necessary in Ca^{2+}/Mg^{2+}-free Earle's balanced salt solution (EBSS) from any of the major suppliers (Gibco or Flow). In the following sections (2.1.1–2.1.3) concentrations given are for stock solutions, weights are approximate, volumes referred to are useful aliquot sizes for storage, and code numbers are those current for Sigma reagents.

2.1.1 Disaggregation buffer stocks

You will need to prepare:

- 25 mg/ml trypsin Type 1 (T-8003) 100 μl
- 4 mg/ml soybean trypsin inhibitor (T-9003) 2 ml

- 200 U/ml deoxyribonuclease I (DNase) (D-4527) 800 μl
- 'solution 4' 800 μl aliquots of bovine serum albumin (BSA) fraction V (A-8022) (150 mg/ml), 0.7 M glucose (0.13 g/ml), 75 mM $MgSO_4.7H_2O$ (18 mg/ml)
- 300 mM $MgSO_4.7H_2O$ (72 mg/ml)

2.1.2 Media stocks

The aliquot sizes given here are for small scale cultures using 20 ml of medium.
Prepare:

- 29 mg/ml glutamine 200 μl. At this concentration glutamine will precipitate when aliquots are thawed. Redissolving the glutamine is quick and does not compromise the cell culture.
- 1.65 M glucose (0.30 g/ml) 400 μl
- 2.45 M KCl (0.18 g/ml) 200 μl
- fetal calf serum (FCS, undiluted) 2 ml. We have found little difference between batches of FCS for granule cell growth. Granule cells will also grow in various serum replacements/extenders such as Nu-Serum when these are used at similar final concentrations to FCS (10%).
- 1.5 mg/ml insulin from bovine pancreas (I–5500) 400 μl. At this concentration the insulin is in suspension. High levels of insulin can replace FCS and will allow granule cell growth, although see Section 4.
- 5 mg/ml and 5000 U/ml penicillin–streptomycin solution 100 μl, or 5 mg/ml gentamycin solution 100 μl. Penicillin–streptomycin is routinely used but gentamycin is also tolerated well by granule cells in serum-containing media. Do not use gentamycin in serum-free media. Both solutions are widely available commercially.

2.1.3 Poly-lysine stock

See Section 2.1.

2.2 Buffers and media for cell culture

Immediately prior to making the cell culture, prepare the following solutions. To do this you will need:

- stock solutions described in section 2.1
- 30 ml sterile Universal containers (plastic or glass)
- EBSS
- BSA
- minimal essential medium (Eagle's modified) with Earle's salts (any major supplier)
- sterile 10 ml pipettes

- sterile 0.2 μm filters (Minisarts—see below), and 10 and 20 ml syringes (these need to be clean but not necessarily sterile)

Four solutions need to be prepared for the disaggregation of the cerebellar tissue into a single cell suspension. We refer to these as buffers A–D. In addition, poly-D-lysine, for coating culture substrates, and tissue culture medium must also be prepared.

(a) Buffer A—trypsinization buffer
- 10 ml EBSS
- 200 μl solution 4
- 100 μl trypsin

(b) Buffer B—inhibitor buffer
- 9 ml EBSS
- 200 μl solution 4
- 1 ml trypsin inhibitor
- 200 μl deoxyribonuclease
- 200 μl $MgSO_4$

(c) Buffer C—disaggregation buffer
- 8 ml EBSS
- 200 μl solution 4
- 1 ml trypsin inhibitor
- 600 μl deoxyribonuclease
- 200 μl $MgSO_4$

(d) Buffer D—gradient buffer
- 10 ml EBSS
- 400 mg bovine serum albumin powder
- 200 μl solution 4

(e) Culture medium
- 18 ml minimal essential medium (Eagle's modified) with Earle's salts
- 2 ml FCS or 400 μl insulin or 2 ml serum replacement/extender
- 200 μl glutamine
- 400 μl glucose
- 200 μl KCl
- 100 μl antibiotic (penicillin–steptomycin or gentamycin)

(f) Poly-D-lysine
- 9 ml double distilled deionized water
- 1 mg/ml poly-D-lysine

(g) Filtration. The above volumes of media and buffers are ideally suited for preparation in 30 ml Universal containers. The non-sterile solutions should then be sterile filtered into fresh, sterile Universals using mini filters. We have found that Sartorius Minisart NML 0.2 µm filters (SM 16534) are ideal for this purpose. Other similar filters are either too small to sit easily on to the Universal or have poor capacities. No ethylene oxide toxicity problems have been noted with these filters. Two filters are all that are required if one uses one for buffers A–D in sequence then the medium, and the second for the poly-D-lysine addition. If larger quantities of medium are required, say above 60 ml, then a third filter specifically for the medium can be used to prevent clogging. After filtration, buffers and media are transferred to a 5% CO_2, 37 °C incubator for 2–4 h to equilibrate. Buffer D contains a high BSA concentration and will appear very acidic (yellow) even after 4 h in the incubator. However it does not appear to have a marked effect on the granule cells.

Protocol 1. Granule cell culture

With practice the culture can be completed in 1.25 h. All instruments should be autoclaved and/or flame sterilized. Other equipment, e.g. the Teflon disc can be scrubbed with 70% ethanol.

Equipment and reagents

- Rat pups six to eight-days-old
- Shaking water-bath at 37 °C
- Two pairs of watchmaker's forceps
- One pair of coarse forceps for handling glass Pasteur pipettes
- One medium sized pair of scissors
- At least two siliconized plugged long-form glass Pasteur pipettes, autoclaved—to siliconize the pipettes immerse them in Repelcote (dimethyldicholorosilane) for 30–60 min ensuring that the cotton wool plug is inserted later: after drying a residue of HCl is left on the pipettes but this is removed during autoclaving
- Sterile 15 ml conical test-tubes and a suitable holder
- Bench centrifuge with rotors for 15 ml conical tubes
- Haemocytometer

- Trypan blue 0.2% in phosphate-buffered saline
- 0–200 µl and 0–1 ml Gilson pipettes or equivalent with corresponding sterile tips (individually wrapped or autoclaved in racks)
- Sterile 10 ml plugged pipettes
- A **thick**-walled Pasteur pipette teat
- Sterile graduated plastic Pasteur pipettes
- One small sized pair of fine pointed scissors
- One small spatula
- One single edged razor blade
- Two or three pieces of either flat scintered glass or roughened Perspex 4 cm x 10 cm
- 20 cm square piece of aluminium foil
- One approx. 3 cm diameter Teflon disc

A.   *Tissue dissection*

1. Kill the rat pups by careful cervical dislocation and then remove their heads using the larger pair of scissors (*Figure 1a*). Place the heads on the rectangle of aluminium foil, scrubbed down with 70% ethanol in a sterile hood. Spray the heads with 70% ethanol.

2. Hold one of the heads dorsal surface uppermost so its rear cut sur-

face is visible. Locate the top of the spinal cord (now seen in cross-section, see *Figure 1b*) and insert one tip of the small fine pointed scissors holding them horizontally at an 8 o'clock position. Keeping the scissor point pressed against the left side (top in *Figure 1b*) of the spinal column cut forwards below the left ear (*Figure 1c*). Now cut over the skull to the other ear (*Figure 1d*). You will be cutting into the cerebral cortices but these are not required in this preparation. Peel the skull over from left to right and trim it away (*Figure 1e*). If there is resistance to peeling, check the first cut from spinal cord to left ear is complete. You have now exposed the dorsal surface of the brain (*Figure 1f*). Visible are the developing pons and medulla, cerebellum, inferior and superior colliculi, and (somewhat damaged) cerebral cortices.

3. Pull away the developing pontine area using the small spatula by inserting it along the division between it and the cerebellum (white dotted line in *Figure 2a*).

4. Similarly divide the cerebellum and underlying tissue from the colliculi by following the cleft between the structures (dotted line in *Figure 2b*).

5. Lift out the cerebellum and underlying material and place on the scintered glass blocks or roughened Perspex.

6. Repeat for the remaining heads.

7. Remove the cerebella from the underlying tissue and clean off the meninges as far as is possible. Use the watchmaker's forceps to pull away the pale, white, developing medullary region from the more heavily vascularized, invaginated cerebellum (*Figure 3*). Use the fine forceps to roll the cerebella lengthwise over the dry rough surface. This tears away most of the meninges but cannot remove all of it due to the involuted structure of the cerebellum. Transfer the cleaned cerebella to the flat Teflon disc for mincing.

8. Mince the tissue using a single edged razor blade with two passes at 90° to each other at approx. 0.5 mm intervals. Transfer the minced tissue using the small spatula to 10 ml buffer A for the start of disaggregation.

Note: It is important not to waste time over the dissection, cleaning, and chopping stages. Desiccation and overhandling of the cerebella can cause much cell damage. For the first few attempts at this method place the cerebella (with underlying tissue) as they are removed from the heads into a Petri dish containing a sterile buffered solution such as EBSS or PBS until all are ready for further manipulation.

B.   Tissue disaggregation

1. Transfer buffer A containing the chopped tissue to the shaking water-bath at 37 °C. Leave to shake vigorously for 15 min during this

Protocol 1 *Continued*

trypsinization step. The exact details of this step can be varied. For example a small, glass conical flask can be used instead of a Universal container and indeed may give better results. Successful cultures can also be prepared by performing the trypsinization simply in the CO_2 incubator with/out shaking. Again what is important is consistency of method.

2. At the end of trypsinization the tissue pieces will probably have become embedded in partially opaque, sputum-like jelly of DNA released from damaged cells. The advantage of trypsinizing in a shaking water-bath is that the mechanical shear forces reduce DNA gel formation significantly and thus improve enzymic access to the tissue.

3. Transfer 10 ml buffer B containing the trypsin inhibitor and deoxyribonuclease into the buffer A/tissue mixture. The DNA jelly will now dissolve due to the action of the deoxyribonuclease. Two or three gentle inversions of the mixture will assist this. Sometimes the DNA may not dissolve and this makes tissue disaggregation very difficult or impossible. Addition of further DNase and/or its cofactor magnesium is rarely of any assistance and the culture may have to be abandoned at this point. In our experience the presence of excess DNA is due to poor inhibition of the trypsin in buffer A (and presumably proteases released from damaged cells). This problem can be largely overcome by raising the trypsin inhibitor concentration. This modification has eliminated the problem of excessive DNA gel formation.

4. Once the DNA has been dissolved the solution and tissue should be divided equally into two sterile screw-top 15 ml conical centrifuge tubes and centrifuged at room temperature for 10 sec at 180 g to pellet the tissue chunks.

5. Discard the supernatant and gently resuspend the tissue pieces in 1.5 ml of buffer C per tube.

6. Disaggregate the tissue pieces into a single cell suspension by trituration using siliconized, sterile, long-form glass Pasteur pipettes. This step is critical and will be developed only through practice. An apparently trivial point is important here. A thick-walled pipette teat is essential to provide the right degree of force for trituration. In our laboratory these are guarded jealously. Trituration is achieved by firmly pressing the tip of the pipette (which must not be chipped or cracked) to the bottom of the conical tube. Steadily and slowly draw up all the contents of the tubes hearing the tissue between tip and tube. At a similar pace expel the solution back into the tube. This represents one pass. Repeat at this pace for three or four more

passes. Complete 10–12 more passes at a higher rate and force but still treating the tissue sympathetically. At the end of this stage almost all of the tissue should be disaggregated into a single cell suspension, with a few pieces left. After 1–2 min settling time remove the supernatants and transfer them to two fresh conical tubes. If one does not need the maximum cell yield from the tissue then add 1.25 ml of buffer C to each of the supernatants and pass to step 7. The remaining tissue pieces can be further disaggregated by the addition of l.25 ml of buffer C to each of the original tubes and trituration as before. Do not feel compelled to disaggregate every last piece of tissue, the more resistant material is often meningeal lining which is not required. After this second trituration step transfer the two new supernatants to the two original supernatants.

7. The two tubes of pooled supernatants contain the cell suspension and some debris. To reduce the amount of debris they must now be centrifuged through buffer D—which constitutes a 4% BSA gradient. Using a graduated plastic Pasteur pipette underlay each of the two supernatants with 2 ml of buffer D. Place the tip of the pipette just off the bottom of the centrifuge tube and gently expel the BSA solution. With care this yields a two-step gradient which should be centrifuged at 180 g for 5 min.

8. Discard the supernatant from the two centrifuge tubes leaving behind a loose cell pellet. Gentle flicking of the bottom of the tube is often sufficient to resuspend the cells in the small amount of buffer present. Add 1–2 ml of buffer C (or Ca^{2+}/Mg^{2+}-free EBSS) to the resuspended pellet; record the total volume of cell suspension achieved.

9. Using a Gilson pipette (or similar) and a sterile tip remove 50 µl of the cell suspension and mix this gently with an equal volume of trypan blue solution. Count the number of viable (unstained, bright) cells using a haemocytometer. A normal cell yield would be between $5–10 \times 10^6$ viable cells per animal used. Cell yields vary depending on the age of the animal and number of pups used. Paradoxically, increasing the number of rats often reduces the cell yield per animal. We normally use three to six animals. Eight-day pups will yield more cells than six-day-old animals but tend to give more debris and dead cells. A good cell preparation should have in the region of 10% dead cells, i.e. stained by trypan blue. For consistency, particularly due to the significant developmental changes that occur in the cerebellum between six and eight days, one should attempt to use animals of the same age for each cell preparation.

10. Again using a Gilson pipette (or similar) and a sterile tip remove an appropriate amount of cell suspension for your requirements and add it to the cell culture medium. Our routine seeding density is 1000

Protocol 1 *Continued*

viable cells/mm² of culture vessel surface. This equates to approx. 10^6 cells/35 mm dish. Each dish contains 3 ml of medium so sufficient cell suspension must be added to the culture medium to give a final concentration of 0.33 million cells/ml.

Note: It is important to realize that whilst perfectly acceptable granule cell cultures may be prepared using variations on this schedule, consistency of method is essential to avoid subtle changes in granule cell development and survival.

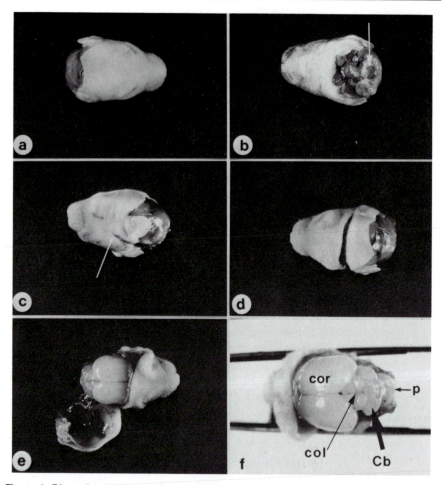

Figure 1. Dissection to expose the cerebellum. (b) *Arrow* marks the point on the circumference of the spinal cord for the first cut. (c) *Arrow* indicates its extent. Cor = cortex; col = colliculi (*arrow* marks the centre of the four elements); p = developing pons; Cb = cerebellum.

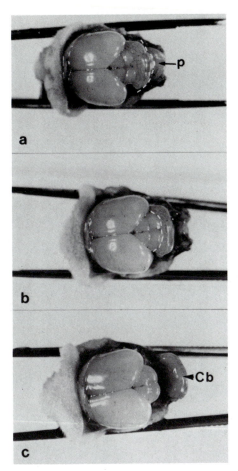

Figure 2. Stages in the removal of the cerebellum. (a) The dotted line indicates where to divide the cerebellum from the pons area. (b) Demonstrates the border between cerebellum and colliculi. (c) The cerebellum (Cb) and underlying tissue have been pulled away from the colliculi ready for removal.

3. Granule cells in culture

Granule cells grow very rapidly *in vitro* and many will produce processes within minutes or hours of plating (*Figure 4*). They can readily be identified in cultures by their small round cell bodies of 8 µm diameter and the presence of one or two neurites. On a cell number basis granule cells will constitute in the region of 90–95% of the cell population. To prevent overgrowth of the cultures grown in FCS containing media with non-neuronal cells a mitotic inhibitor such as fluorodeoxyuridine (80 µM) should be added to the medium after one day. Serum-free media, e.g. with insulin replacing FCS do not need

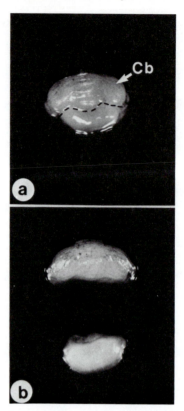

Figure 3. Cleaning the cerebellum. The underlying tissue is separated from the cerebellum (Cb) using fine forceps to split the material along the dotted line.

this addition. Such cultures often appear 'dirty' partly due to increased cell death but also due to the lack of macrophage activity. Insulin-containing medium will support granule cell growth but it is probably suboptimal and an increased plating density of $1.5–2.0 \times 10^6$ cells/35 mm dish improves cell survival. Other cells found within the cultures are: astrocytes of at least two morphologies, flattened (Type I-like) and multiprocessed Type II-like), a few fibroblast-like cells, multiprocessed GABAergic interneurons, large oligodendrocytes with numerous processes possessing bulbous expansions or thin sheets of membrane, macrophages, and a few large, phase-bright non-processed Purkinje cells.

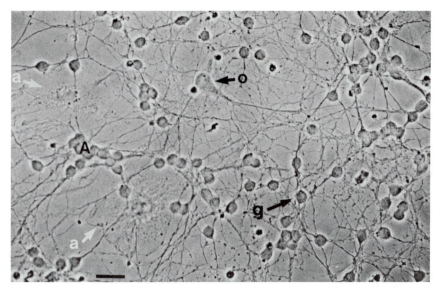

Figure 4. A two to three day *in vitro* granule cell culture. Numerous granule cell perikarya can be seen (g) amid a meshwork of fine processes. Some neurons have aggregated (A). Non-neuronal cells such as probable astrocytes (a) and oligodendro-cytes (o) are also present. Scale bar = 20 μm. Figure courtesy of Dr S. Przyborski.

References

1. Currie, D. N., Dutton, G. R., and Cohen, J. (1979). *Experientia*, **35,** 345.
2. Dutton, G. R., Currie, D. N., and Tear, K. T. (1981). *J. Neurosci. Meth.*, **3,** 421.

2

Cerebellar Purkinje neurons

SUSANA COHEN-CORY

1. Introduction

Cultured Purkinje neurons provide a good model for studying the roles of intrinsic neuronal properties, environmental signals, and cell–cell interactions during development and differentiation. Some of the cellular events that lead to the morphological and functional differentiation of Purkinje neurons, as well as the ontogeny and organization of the cerebellar circuitry are known. Moreover, due to the feasibility of electrophysiological and pharmacological manipulations in culture, Purkinje neurons have provided an excellent system for studying the development of neuronal electrical activity and transmitter sensitivity (1,2). The roles that neural activity, hormones, neurotrophic factors, and cell–cell interactions play during Purkinje cell development are now beginning to be elucidated (3--6).

The developing and mature Purkinje neurons are a biochemically and anatomically heterogeneous neuronal population. During early development, certain clusters of Purkinje neurons express biochemical markers that others express at a very low level or not at all. This apparent early biochemical heterogeneity may be due the difference in the timing of development among Purkinje neurons from the distinct cerebellar areas (7,8). Conversely, for some cellular markers expression becomes gradually restricted to subsets of Purkinje neurons as development proceeds (9). In the mature cerebellum, biochemically and physiologically distinct Purkinje neurons organize in parasagittal bands. Mature Purkinje neurons are inhibitory and use gamma-aminobutyric acid (GABA) as their major neurotransmitter. Thus, these neurons synthesize GABA and express the neurotransmitter synthesizing enzyme glutamic acid decarboxylase (GAD). During early postnatal development, Purkinje neurons transiently express several acetylcholine related enzymes, as well as muscarinic acetylcholine receptors. In addition to these neurotransmitter related markers, Purkinje neurons can be identified by their high expression of second messenger related enzymes and receptor proteins like cyclic GMP-dependent protein kinase and inositol trisphosphate (IP$_3$) receptor. One abundantly expressed protein by both developing and mature Purkinje neurons is the vitamin D-dependent calcium binding protein

Calbindin D$_{28K}$. Calbindin serves as an excellent marker to identify Purkinje neurons in culture, since it is highly expressed in most early developing Purkinje neurons and is not expressed by any other neuronal type within the cerebellar cortex (10).

2. Nutrient media

2.1. Nutrient medium supplemented with serum

The use of a nutrient media supplemented with serum (*Protocol 1*) provides a rich environment for the growth and differentiation of Purkinje neurons in culture. Maintaining embryonic rat and mouse cerebellar cell cultures in serum-containing medium fosters the survival and differentiation of Purkinje neurons by allowing the survival of both neurons and non-neuronal cells. Interactions between neurons and glia in culture are important for the normal differentiation of the Purkinje cell population. Survival and differentiation can be further enhanced by the addition of hormones, growth factors, or depolarizing agents to the culture medium (3,4,11). Purkinje neurons can be maintained in culture media supplemented with serum for up to 10–12 days in the absence of antimitotic agents. This affords a reasonable time window in which to study the development and response of this neuronal population to different exogenous agents. Major limitations with the use of serum-supplemented medium are the limited control of components present in the undefined medium, and the unrestricted proliferation of non-neuronal cells after two weeks in culture that can reduce the long-term survival of the Purkinje cell population. There are several ways to prevent the effects of unrestricted non-neuronal proliferation and competition for nutrients. One is to reduce the concentration of serum after the first three days in culture by replacing the serum-containing medium with fresh media prepared with lower concentrations of serum (2% or 5%). Alternatively, one can treat cultures with antimitotic agents such as fluorodeoxyuridine five days after plating, at which time a non-confluent monolayer of support cells is already present. Finally, cultures can be grown in a chemically defined, serum-free medium after the initial plating in serum-supplemented medium. The composition of the serum-supplemented nutrient medium is: minimal essential medium with Earle's salts, 2 mM glutamine, 6 mg/ml glucose, 10% heat inactivated horse serum, 0.5 U/ml penicillin, 0.5 µg/ml streptomycin.

Protocol 1. Preparation of nutrient medium containing serum

Equipment and reagents

- Pre-sterilized, disposable plastic pipettes (5 ml and 10 ml capacity)
- Pre-sterilized, disposable plastic culture tubes (15 ml and 50 ml capacity)
- Sterile syringe filter units (Gelman Scientific, Acrodisc 4192)
- Pre-sterilized disposable plastic syringes

- Eagles minimal essential medium with Earle's salts (MEM), supplemented with 2 mM L-glutamine (Gibco, 320–1095AG)
- D (+) Glucose (Sigma, G7021)
- Horse serum (Gibco, 200–6050AG)—heat inactivate in a 56 °C water-bath for 30 min: prepare 10 ml aliquots in sterile plastic tubes and store at –20 °C until use
- Penicillin–streptomycin stock solution: 5000 U/ml penicillin and 5 mg/ml streptomycin in 0.9% sodium chloride (Sigma P3539)—prepare a 50 U penicillin/50 µg streptomycin working solution by diluting 1 : 100 in sterile-filtered tc-H$_2$O: divide into aliquots and store at –20 °C

Method

1. For 100 ml of media, weigh out 0.6 g of glucose and transfer to a sterile plastic test-tube.

2. With a sterile plastic pipette, transfer 10 ml of MEM to the tube containing glucose, and dissolve by gently mixing. Sterile filter through a 0.22 µm filter unit into a sterile bottle containing 80 ml of MEM.

3. Thaw a 10 ml aliquot of heat inactivated horse serum and transfer to the MEM/glucose solution with a sterile plastic 10 ml pipette.

4. Add 1 ml of the 50 U penicillin/ 50 µg streptomycin working solution to the media and mix gently.

5. The media is ready for use, and should be stored at 4 °C for no more than one week.

2.2 Chemically defined, serum-free medium

The use of a chemically defined, serum-free medium is recommended for studies in which better control of the factors present in the nutrient medium is desired. This is especially important in studies in which the presence of serum components may mask or alter the effects of agents of study. One advantage of the use of chemically defined serum-free medium is that by preventing unrestricted proliferation of non-neuronal cells, longer survival of the Purkinje cell population may be achieved. In this medium, Purkinje neurons can survive for more than a month, provided they are initially plated at a relatively high density. One limitation to growing cells in serum-free medium is that dendritic differentiation is maintained in an arrested state during the first two weeks in culture. This may be due to the lack of nutrient or differentiation factors that are otherwise present in mixed neuron–glial cultures in serum-containing media (3–5). A new methodological approach directed to study the role of cellular interactions between purified populations of Purkinje cells (purified by density gradient centrifugation and immunopanning) and other neuronal and non-neuronal populations in culture, has recently been published (6). The composition of the serum-free medium described below is a modification of that described by Fischer (12); basal medium Eagle with Earle's salts, supplemented with 2 mM L-glutamine, 1 mg/ml bovine serum albumin, 10 µg/ml insulin, 0.1 nM thyroxine, 0.1 mg/ml transferrin, 30 nM selenium, 0.25% glucose, 0.5 U/ml penicillin, 0.5 µg/ml streptomycin.

Protocol 2. Preparation of chemically defined, serum-free medium

Equipment and reagents
- Basal medium Eagle with Earle's salts (BME) supplemented with 2 mM L-glutamine (Gibco, 320–1015AG)
- Bovine serum albumin (BSA, Sigma, A3294)
- Insulin (Sigma, I6634)
- L-Thyroxine (Sigma, T1775)
- Transferrin (Sigma, T7786)
- Sodium selenite (Sigma, S5261)
- D (+) Glucose (Sigma, G7021)
- Penicillin–streptomycin working solution: 50 U penicillin/ 50 µg streptomycin (see *Protocol 1*)

Method

1. Make a 1 mM thyroxine stock solution by dissolving 1.54 mg of thyroxine in 200 µl of a 70% ethanol/0.1 M sodium hydroxide solution, and diluting to 2 ml with sterile tc-H_2O. Prepare a second stock solution of 10 µM thyroxine in tc-H_2O and store at 4 °C. Make a 0.1 µM thyroxine working solution in tc-H_2O.

2. Prepare a 3 mM sodium selenite stock solution by dissolving 1 mg of sodium selenite in 2 ml of sterile tc-H_2O. Make a 30 µM working solution by diluting 1 : 100 in tc-H_2O.

3. For 100 ml of media, dissolve 1 mg of insulin in 200 µl of sterile filtered 0.01 M HCl solution.

4. Combine 10 mg of transferrin, 100 mg of BSA, and 250 mg of glucose in a 10 ml tube, and dissolve with 10 ml of BME.

5. With a sterile 1 ml pipette, transfer the insulin solution (step 3) into the tube containing transferrin–BSA–glucose in BME and mix. Filter sterilize through a 0.22 µm filter unit, and collect the filtrate in a sterile bottle containing 90 ml of BME.

6. With sterile pipettes, transfer 0.1 ml of the 0.1 µM thyroxine and 0.1 ml of the 30 µM selenium working solutions to the medium and mix.

7. Add 1 ml of the penicillin–streptomycin working solution and mix gently.

8. The serum-free medium is ready to use and should be stored at 4 °C for no more than two to three weeks.

3. Dissection and tissue preparation

3.1 Optimal stage for growing Purkinje neurons

Success in growing Purkinje neurons is highly dependent on the developmental stage at which the neurons are plated. Optimal survival is obtained when cultures are prepared from embryos one to two days after the peak in Purkinje cell birth. Thus, maximal survival and differentiation of rat Purkinje neurons is achieved by plating dissociated cerebellar cells obtained from embryos of 15 to 17 days of gestation (gestation period is 22 days). Reduced survival is obtained if cultures are prepared from embryos of more than 19 days gestation.

While the methods described in this chapter have been optimized for culturing embryonic rat cerebellar Purkinje neurons, the same methods can be applied to the growth of mouse Purkinje neurons. In the mouse embryo, Purkinje neurons cease to divide at about the 12th to 13th day of gestation (the gestation period is 18 days). Thus, the optimal stage for culturing is at embryonic days 14 to 16, although Purkinje neurons can survive in cultures prepared from postnatal day one mouse cerebella.

3.2 Removal of embryos

This procedure is described in full in Chapter 3.

3.3 Cerebellar dissection from embryonic rat

Figure 1 in Chapter 1 is a further guide to this dissection.

Protocol 3.   Cerebellar dissection

1. With a pair of small serrated forceps and scissors, pull back the fetal or neonatal skin covering the head and expose the skull. Gently cut open the skull along the lateral edges and along the midline fissure. Take care not to damage the brain and cerebellar tissues underneath. Cut the bone and cartilage caudal to the cerebellum, at the level of the rostral spinal cord, and pull open the skull to expose the brain.

2. With a pair of curved forceps, pull out the rostral part of the brain, at the level of the olfactory bulbs. With the small scissors cut the optic nerves from the ventral midbrain and release the brain with the cerebellum intact from the skull.

3. Place each brain in a 100 mm glass Petri dish with PBS. Separate the cerebellum from surrounding brain tissue under the dissecting microscope. With a pair of scalpel blades, unfold the dorsal midbrain and dissect to expose the cerebellum (*Figure 1a*).

4. Make a cut at the level of the caudal midbrain to dissect out from the rest of the brain (*Figure 1b*). With a second cut dissect away the spinal cord laying caudally (*Figure 1c*). Flip the cross-section so that the brain-stem can be removed (see *Figure 1d*). Trim the remaining tissue so as to collect only the cerebellar tissue medial to the cerebellar peduncles (see *Figure 1e*).

Protocol 3 *Continued*

5. Place all pieces of cerebellum in a sterile glass 35 mm Petri dish containing enough nutrient medium to completely cover the tissue. With a pair of fine forceps, carefully peel off the meningeal tissue overlying the cerebellum (the meningeal sheet may peel off when dissecting the cerebellum from surrounding tissues).

6. Pool the clean cerebellar tissue from 10 to 20 embryos or pups in a fresh small glass Petri dish containing 2 ml of nutrient media, and mince the tissue into 0.5–1.0 mm pieces with the scalpel blades.

7. Collect the minced tissue in nutrient media with a long-necked Pasteur pipette, and transfer to a sterile plastic 15 ml centrifuge tube.

8. Dissociate immediately by mechanical dissociation or by enzymatic digestion with papain (see *Protocols 4* and *5*).

4. Tissue dissociation, plating densities, and conditions for cell growth

4.1 Mechanical and enzymatic tissue dissociation

The dissociation of cerebellar tissue into single cells can be accomplished by either mechanical dissociation or enzymatic treatment followed by mechanical dissociation. Simple mechanical dissociation is recommended for studies in which little disturbance of the membrane receptor proteins is desired. Both fetal and neonatal cerebellar tissues can be easily and rapidly dissociated by trituration with a Pasteur pipette, while preserving cell integrity and allowing survival in culture. The dissociation of neurons by enzymatic treatment with mechanical trituration leads to a better recovery of neurons, and hence to better survival. Both mechanical trituration and enzymatic digestion followed by mechanical trituration yield neurons that retain their ability to express normal biochemical and morphological characteristics in culture. Enzymatic treatments with papain or trypsin have been used successfully to dissociate embryonic as well as neonatal cerebellar cells. A method that uses papain for the dissociation (13) is presented in this chapter.

Protocol 4. Mechanical dissociation

1. With a long-necked sterile Pasteur pipette, transfer the minced cerebellar tissue in nutrient media to a sterile 15 ml conical tube.

2. Gently triturate the tissue by pipetting up and down with the Pasteur pipette. Triturate the tissue by pipetting eight to ten times, until the tissue breaks into smaller pieces. Disperse the small clumps of tissue into single cells by repeating the trituration with a flame-polished Pasteur pipette, the bore of which has been narrowed to about one-third

of its original size. Mechanically dissociate the cerebellar cells by triturating eight to ten times.

3. Mix the cell suspension gently with a new sterile long-necked Pasteur
   pipette, and withdraw one drop of this cell suspension to determine
   cell yield and efficiency of dispersion (see section 4.2).

Protocol 5. Enzymatic dissociation using papain

Equipment and reagents

- Horizontal shaker
- Automatic pipettor
- Table-top clinical centrifuge
- Papain, from *Carica papaya*, crystalline suspension (Boehringer Mannheim, 108 014)
- Cysteine–HCl (Sigma, C-7880)

- Bicarbonate-buffered salt solution (BBSS): 25 mM sodium bicarbonate, 125 mM sodium chloride, 3 mM potassium chloride, 0.5 mM sodium phosphate pH 7.4, 0.25 mM calcium chloride, 1 mM sodium pyruvate, 16 mM glucose, 0.01% aqueous phenol red

Method

1. Prepare a working solution of papain by dissolving 8 mg of cysteine–
   HCl in 10 ml of BBSS in a sterile plastic test-tube immediately before
   use. Mix the papain stock suspension thoroughly and add 7 U of
   enzyme/ml of BBSS–cysteine mix. Resuspend and adjust the pH of the
   solution by placing the tube in the humidified CO_2 incubator for 15–20
   min to solubilize.

2. Sterile filter through a 0.22 μm syringe filter unit and collect in a sterile
   plastic 15 ml centrifuge tube.

3. With a sterile Pasteur pipette, transfer the minced cerebellar tissue to
   the tube containing the papain. Transfer as little nutrient media as
   possible. Cap the tube, place on the shaker, and rock gently (100
   r.p.m.) for 20–30 min at 37 °C.

4. Sediment the tissue by centrifugation at 1000 r.p.m. for 5 min. With
   a sterile 10 ml plastic pipette, carefully remove the papain solution
   and discard. Rinse the tissue with 10 ml of sterile filtered PBS (room
   temperature).

5. Sediment the tissue by centrifugation and discard the PBS solution.
   Take care not to disturb the tissue pellet.

6. Repeat the wash step twice and carefully pipette 2 ml of serum-
   supplemented nutrient medium into the tube.

7. Disperse the tissue clumps into single cells by gentle trituration with a
   flame-polished Pasteur pipette.

8. Pipette five to six times, or until clumps are no longer seen.

Protocol 5 *Continued*

9. Mix the cell suspension gently with a new Pasteur pipette and with-draw one drop of the cell suspension to determine cell yield and efficiency of dissociation (see section 4.2).

4.2 Determination of cell yields and plating density

Cell yield varies between dissociation methods and between experiments. It is therefore necessary to determine cell yield and calculate the number of cells per volume for each experiment prior to plating. Medium to moderate density cultures are obtained by plating 1×10^5 cells/cm^2 in either 35 mm tissue culture dishes or well plates. The final density of plating is 1×10^6 cell/35 mm dish. Immediately after plating, place cultures in the 37 °C humidified CO_2 incubator.

4.3 Conditions for cell growth

Purkinje neurons grow optimally at 37 °C in a 5% CO_2, humidified incubator. The culture media can be replaced as often as every four days or as late as every week to replenish nutrients. When replacing culture media, it is important to replace only one-half of the volume of medium present in each plate, thus allowing for some of the nutrients present in the conditioned medium to remain. When feeding, take care not to detach cells from the substrate. Aspirate the medium gently with a sterile disposable plastic pipette and slowly add fresh nutrient media pre-warmed to 37 °C, to the side of the plate or tissue culture well.

5. Identification of Purkinje neurons

Neuronal cells in culture can be identified by their expression of specific biochemical markers (*Figure 1*). One convenient antigen used for the identification of developing Purkinje neurons in culture is Calbindin D_{28K} (Sigma Immunochemicals), a vitamin-dependent calcium binding protein that, within the cerebellum, is expressed exclusively by Purkinje neurons. Specific antibodies to calbindin and other biochemical markers expressed by Purkinje neurons have been used for the immunostaining and identification of Purkinje neurons in culture. Before immunostaining, cells should be fixed. The type of fixative varies according to the type of antigen to be identified, and the type of antibody to be used. Special care should be given when fixing and immunostaining Purkinje neurons to avoid detachment of cells from the culture substrate. To preserve cells and identify immunocytochemically by the expression of calbindin, cerebellar cultures can be fixed for 3 h at 4 °C in a freshly prepared solution of 4% paraformaldehyde in 0.01 M sodium phosphate buffer pH 7.4.

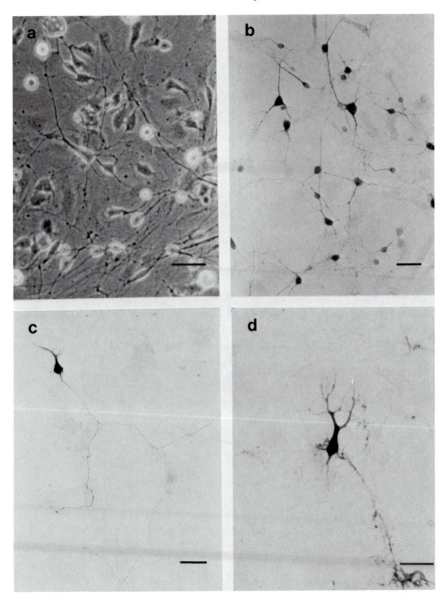

Figure 1. E18 rat cerebellar cells grown in culture for seven days in nutrient medium containing serum, in the presence of 25 mM KCl alone (c), or in combination with nerve growth factor (a, b, and d) (see ref. 3). (a) Phase photomicrograph of cerebellar cells in culture. (b) All cerebellar neurons in culture are visualized by immunostaining with an antibody to neuron-specific enolase (NSE, Sigma Immunochemicals). (c) and (d) Purkinje neurons are visualized by immunostaining with an antibody to calbindin. Note the enhanced Purkinje cell dendritic differentiation in cultures grown in the presence of trophic factors (d). Scale bar, 50 μm.

Susana Cohen-Cory

Acknowledgements

This work was developed in the laboratories of Dr Ira Black at the UMDNJ-Robert Wood Johnson Medical School, and Dr Torsten Wiesel at the Rockefeller University, and was supported by the NIH and the Lucille P. Markey Charitable Trust. I thank Drs Ira Black and Cheryl Dreyfus for advice, and Dr Howard Mount for helpful comments.

References

1. Gruol, D. L. (1983). *Brain Res.*, **263,** 223.
2. Yusaki, M. and Mikoshiba, K. (1992). *J. Neurosci.*, **12,** 4253.
3. Cohen-Cory, S., Dreyfus, C. F., and Black, I. B. (1991). *J. Neurosci.*, **11,** 462.
4. Mount, T. J., Dreyfus, C. F., and Black, I. B. (1993). *J. Neurosci.*, **13,** 3173.
5. Lindhom, D., Castréu, E., Tsoulfas, P., Kolbeck, R., Berzaghi, M. D. P., Leingartner, A. (1993). *J. Cell Biol.*, **122,** 443.
6. Baptista, C. A., Hatten, M. E., Blazeski, R., and Mason, C. A. (1994). *Neuron*, **12,** 243.
7. Ito, M. (1984). *The cerebellum and neural control.* Raven Press, New York.
8. Wassef, M. and Sotelo, C. (1984). *Neuroscience*, **13,** 1217.
9. Leclerc, N., Gravel, C., and Hawkes, R. (1988). *J. Comp. Neurol.*, **273,** 399.
10. Christakos, S., Rhoten, W. B., and Feldman, S. C. (1987) In *Methods in enzymology* (ed. A.R. Means), Vol. 139, pp. 534–51. Academic Press, San Diego.
11. Audinat, E., Knopfel, T., and Gahwiler, B. H. (1991). *J. Physiol.*, **430,** 297.
12. Fischer, G. (1982). *Neurosci. Lett.*, **28,** 325.
13. Burous O'Malley, M. and MacLeish, P. R. (1993). *J. Neurosci. Meth.*, **47,** 61.

3

Nigral and striatal neurons

ROGER BARKER and ALAN JOHNSON

1. Introduction

This chapter describes simple and reliable methods for the culture of dissociated nigral and striatal neurons. We give an accurate definition of the conditions required for the survival of these cells. These data may have implications for studies on neural development as well as those concerned with neuro-degeneration. In this last respect two of the commonly encountered yet major neurodegenerative diseases of the CNS are Parkinson's disease (PD) and Huntington's Chorea (HC), which predominantly affect the dopaminer-gic nigral and GABAergic striatal neurons respectively (1,2). This coupled to the use of these cells for intracerebral transplantation (3), has led to a large number of *in vitro* studies involving these neuronal populations (see *Table 1* and *2*). There is, however, no universally adopted technique although the methods described in this chapter are used in several laboratories and rou-tinely produce reliable results.

2. Equipment

(a) For removing embryos:
- pregnant rat (usually has litter of 10–15)
- jar with cotton wool at base, with screw-lid
- ether
- large blunt tipped scissors
- forceps (not fine)
- Petri dish (5–10 cm diameter) half-filled with Hank's balanced salt solution (HBSS)

(b) For dissecting out embryos:
- small pair of scissors
- fine serrated pair of forceps
- Petri dishes half-filled with HBSS

Table 1. Major *in vitro* studies of dopamine nigral neurons in mouse and rat

Year	Mouse/rat[a]	Embryo age enzyme[b]	Proteolytic procedure[b]	Trituration	Reference
1979	m	E13	—	*	4
1981	m	E14	0.67% T, 35 min	Pasteur	5
1984	m	E13	—	*	6
1986	r	E18	0.25% T, 15 min	Pasteur	7
1986	r	E14	0.2% T, *	*	8
1986	r	E15–16	—	Pasteur	9,10
1987	r	E14	—	*	11
1988	r	E14	—	Pasteur	12
1988	r	E14–15	0.1% T, *	Pasteur	13
1988	m	E13	—	*	14
1988	m	E13–18	—	27 g needle	15
1988	r	E15	—	*	16
1989	r	E14	0.25% T, 5 min	22 g needle	17
1989	r	E15–16	—	Eppendorf	18
1989	r	E15	—	Pasteur/25 g Needle	19
1989	r	E15	0.1% T, 15 min	*	20,21
1990	m	E14	—	*	22
1990	r	E15	—	*	23
1990	r	E15–16	—	Pasteur	24
1991	r	E14	—	*	25
1991	r	E13.5	*T, *	*	26
1991	r	~ E16	0.05% T, 20 min	Pasteur	27
1991	r	E15	—	*	28,29
1991	r	E15	—	22 g needle	30
1991	r	E14.5	0.1% T, 20 min	*	31
1991	r	E14	—	Pasteur	32
1991	r	EI7–postnatal	Papain (9 U/ml)	*	33
1991	r	E14	0.125% T, 20 min	Pasteur	34
1991	r	E16	—	Pasteur	35
1992	r	E15	—	*	36
1992	r	E13–14	0.1% T, 6 min	23 g needle	37

[a]r, rat; m, mouse.
[b]T, trypsin; g, gauge; Pasteur, flamed Pasteur pipette; *, details not given in reference.

(c) For dissecting out ventral mesencephalon:
- dissecting microscope with good light source
- scalpel with standard size 11 blade
- pairs of fine forceps
- pair of microdissection (i.e. spring iridectomy, Dumont No. 5) scissors
- Petri and smaller diameter dishes (2–3 cm) half-filled with HBSS

(d) For preparing cell suspension:
- 10 ml plastic tube with screw-cap

Table 2. Major *in vitro* studies of striatal cells in mouse and rat[a]

Year	Mouse/rat	Embryo age	Proteolytic enzyme	Trituration procedure	Reference
1979	m	E15	—	*	4
1979	r	New-born	—	*	38,39
1981	r	New-born	0.5% T, 14 min	Pasteur	40,41
1982	m	E14	0.67% T, 35 min	Pasteur	5
1984	r	E18	0.08% T, 30 min	Pasteur	42
1986	m	E14–15	—	Pasteur	43
1986	r	E13.5–new-born	—	Pasteur	44
1987	r	E14	—	*	45
1987	r	E18	0.03% T, 60 min	Pasteur	46
1988	r	E17	—	Pasteur	47
1988	m	E14–16	0. 15% T, 60 min	*	48
1989	r	E19–21	—	Pasteur	49
1989	m	E16	—	Pasteur	50
1990	m	E14	—	*	36
1990	r	P0-P6	—	Pasteur	51
1991	r	E16	—	Pasteur	35
1992	r	Neonatal	—	Pasteur	52

[a] See footnote to *Table 1*.

- trypsin in PBS or HBSS
- DNase in PBS or HBSS
- triturating solution
- 10 ml pipettes
- Pasteur pipettes
- haemocytometer

(e) For plating out dissociated neurons:
- 6-well plastic plates (supplied by Nunc through Gibco-BRL, Paisley Scotland)
- coverslips—usually 22 mm diameter (previously cleaned, sterilized, and coated with polylysine)
- 1 ml pipettes
- poly-D/L-lysine solution
- culture medium

(f) Fixation and immunocytochemistry:
- Petri dishes
- Glyceel or nail varnish
- 1 ml syringe with 21 gauge needle

- PBS
- PBS with 0.2% Triton X-100
- normal goat serum
- antibody to tyrosine hydroxylase
- secondary antibody conjugated to biotin
- streptavidin conjugated to either rhodamine or fluorescein
- small plastic or glass pipettes
- glass microscope slides
- 50% mix of glycerol and PBS

3. Solutions and reagents

All solutions that are used in the preparation of the cell suspension must be sterilized. This can be most easily done by filtering the prepared solutions through a 0.2 μm filter.

(a) Hank's balanced salt solution (HBSS). Supplier: Gibco Ltd, Paisley, Scotland. Use: All tissues are dissected in this solution.

(b) 0.1 M phosphate-buffered saline (PBS). Composed of 8.5 g sodium chloride, 0.4 g dihydrogen sodium phosphate, and 1 g disodium hydrogen phosphate per litre of distilled water; pH 7.2. Use: Main reagent in staining procedure. It is used on its own as a washing solution and is also the main reagent into which other substances used in the staining procedure are dissolved including Triton X-100, paraformaldehyde (both supplied by Merck Ltd, Merck House, Poole, Dorset), and normal goat serum (supplied by Seralab, Crawley Down, Sussex).

(c) Trypsin (1 mg/ml in PBS) solution (porcine, Sigma Cat. No. T0134). Use: Proteolytic digestion of ventral mesencephalon and striatum.

(d) DNase I (10 μg/ml in PBS, Sigma Cat. No. D5025). Use: To prevent cell clumping due to release of DNA from cells damaged in the cell suspension procedure.

(e) Triturating solution. 1 mg/ml BSA, 10 μg/ml DNase I, 0.5 mg/ml soybean trypsin inhibitor (Sigma Cat. No.T9003) in PBS. Use: To inactivate trypsin and allow for mechanical dissociation of the neural tissue to produce final cell suspension.

(f) Poly-L or D-lysine solution (Sigma Cat. No. P0899, M_r 70–150000). Use: It is made up into a 0.01% solution with distilled water and filtered. It is used as a substrate on which the neurons can extend processes on the coverslip (also see Introduction).

(g) Culture medium. Contains: 85% DMEM with high glucose (Imperial Laboratories, Andover, Hampshire), 15% fetal calf serum (Seralab), and fungizone, penicillin, streptomycin (Sigma Chemical Co. Ltd). It is advisable to batch test the fetal calf serum. Use: Neuronal growth medium.

(h) Primary antibody to tyrosine hydroxylase (TH). Supplier: Boehringer Mannheim UK Ltd, Lewes, Sussex. Use: Dilute in PBS/0.2% Triton at a concentration of 1 : 100 with 1% normal goat serum (NGS). It is a monoclonal antibody used to label dopaminergic neurons in ventral mesencephalic cultures.

(i) Secondary antibody for use with mouse monoclonal antibody. Supplier: Caltag, CC Biologicals, Market Harborough, Leicestershire. Used at a dilution of 1 : 100 in PBS/0.2% Triton with 1% NGS.

(j) Streptavidin complex. Supplier: Serotec, Kidlington, Oxford. Use: It binds to the biotinylated secondary antibody and allows visualization of the antibody complex. It is used at a dilution of 1 : 100 in PBS/0.2% Triton with 1% NGS.

(k) PBS/glycerol (50 : 50) mounting solution.

(l) Primary antibody to gamma-aminobutyric acid (GABA). Supplier: Cambridge Research Biochemical Ltd, Northwick, Cheshire. Use: It is a polyclonal antibody used to label striatal cells in culture as about 95% of all striatal cells use this amino acid as a neurotransmitter. It is used at a dilution of 1 : 100 in PBS/0.2% Triton with 1% NGS.

(m) Secondary antibody to GABA. Supplier: Caltag, a biotinylated goat anti-rabbit IgG conjugated to fluorescein isothiocyanate, used at a dilution of 1 : 100 in PBS/0.2% Triton with 1% NGS.

4. Nigral cultures

Equipment and reagents for *Protocols 1–5*. Prior to harvesting embryos set-up the following equipment in a tissue culture hood:

- spirit burner
- small 100 ml beaker with 30 ml of methylated spirits to hold instuments
- small scissors, scalpel, microdissecting scissors, two sets of fine forceps
- large Petri dishes (5–10 cm diameter) half-filled with HBSS
- small Petri dish (2–3 cm diameter) half-filled with HBSS
- 10 ml tube with screw-cap
- 6-well plates (usually two or three)
- coverslips placed out in sterile Petri dishes and covered with 0.01% poly-D/L-lysine solution, so that it forms a meniscus on coverslip
- supply of sterile 10 ml pipettes and Pasteur pipettes

Protocol 1. Killing of pregnant rat and removal of embryos
(see *Figure 1*)

1. The embryonic age of the litter should be known accurately (i.e. use time mated rats), and this should be E14 for nigral cultures, the embryos having a crown-rump length at this age of 10–12 mm (see *Figures 2* and *3*) (3).

2. Asphyxiate pregnant rat with CO_2. Avoid intraperitoneal injection of anaesthetic agents as this can damage embryos.

3. When rat ceases respiration remove and place back down on bench, kill by cervical dislocation.

4. Spray abdomen with methylated spirits.

5. Incise abdomen vertically with scissors to reveal abdominal contents, and then extend incision bilaterally to flanks (*Figure 1a*).

6. Lift string of embryos up with forceps and cut along placental surface to remove from mother (*Figure 1b*), and place into Petri dish half-filled with HBSS.

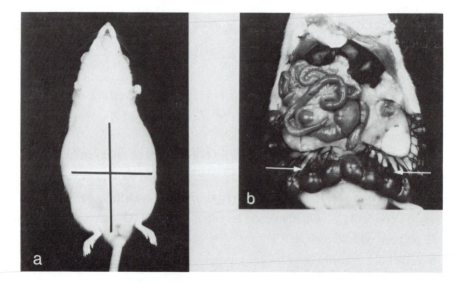

Figure 1. Removal of embryos from mother. (a) Incise abdomen in midline and then extend incision bilaterally to the flanks to reveal abdominal contents including embryos. (b) Remove embryos by incising along placental margin of string of embryos.

Protocol 2. Dissecting out the embryos

1. Return to hood with Petri dish containing embryos.

2. Remove amniotic and chorionic membranes from each embryo by incising along dorsal side of embryonic sac with small scissors. This side is opposite the one along which the embryos were removed from the mother (see *Figure 1b*).

3. The embryonic rats should now appear through cut membranes, although they may require freeing from their placenta by a further cut along the fetal placental surface (see *Figure 1b*).

4. Lift each embryo out and place carefully into a clean Petri dish of HBSS. The best way to achieve this is to rest the embryo across a set of forceps, such that the forceps lie just below the head but above the forelimbs.

5. Wash in this Petri dish and transfer to another Petri dish containing HBSS for dissection of the ventral mesencephalon.

Protocol 3. Dissecting out the ventral mesencephalon (VM) (see *Figure 2*)

1. Place dish containing clean embryos under dissecting microscope.

2. Check crown–rump length of embryo (*Figure 2a*).

3. Make incision with scalpel from eye through mouth up to the ventral mesencephalic flexure (*Figure 2b*).

4. At this point it is advisable to move knife, microdissecting scissors, and forceps so that they rest on a Petri dish lid adjacent to the dissecting microscope.

5. Roll embryo on to its back so allowing forebrain to flop away from brain-stem and reveal base of lateral ventricular system and its continuance in the brain-stem as the 3rd ventricle and central aqueduct (*Figure 2c*).

6. Now with the dissecting scissors cut backwards down either side of the ventricle (CUT 1 in *Figure 2d*), followed by a cut caudally (CUT 2 in *Figure 2d*), followed by a cut at the bottom of the mesencephalic flexure (CUT 3 in *Figure 2d*).

7. The ventral mesencephalic (VM) remnant should now lie free of the rest of the brain.

8. Remove overlying meninges with forceps and place dissected VM into a separate dish of HBSS.

9. This piece resembles a butterfly in shape.

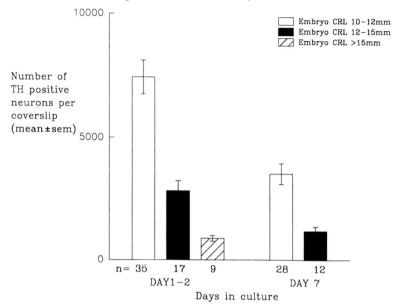

Figure 3. The effects of embryonic age on the survival of dopaminergic nigral neurons *in vitro* (R. Barker, unpublished data). n = number of cultures per time point.

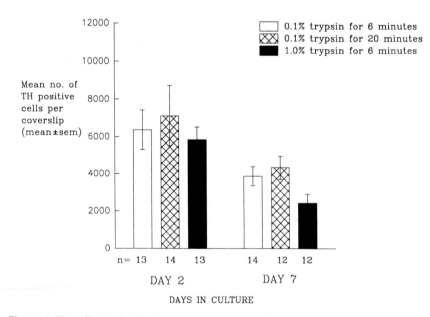

Figure 4. The effects of different trypsinizations on the survival of dopaminergic nigral neurons *in vitro* (R. Barker, unpublished data). n = number of cultures per time point.

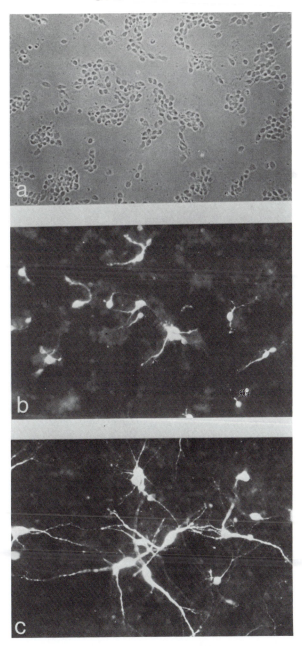

Figure 5. Cultured dopaminergic nigral cells. (a) One-day-old E14 nigral culture showing that the majority of cells are non-dopaminergic as illustrated by the fact that when the same coverslip is stained with an antibody to TH only a few cells stain (b). (c) After eight days in culture the dopaminergic nigral cells have grown both in terms of size and axonal outgrowth (× 170).

5. Striatal cultures

The procedures involved in preparing striatal cultures are very similar to those for nigral cultures. So set-up laminar flow hood as for nigral cultures.

(a) Killing of pregnant rat and removal of embryos is as for nigra cultures, *Protocol 1*. In this case use older embryos, E15–E18 (crown-rump length > 13 mm).

(b) Dissecting out embryos is as for nigral cultures, *Protocol 2*.

Protocol 6. Dissecting out striatal primordia (see *Figure 6*)

1. Strip off skull and meninges to reveal cerebral hemispheres/vesicles by making an incision horizontally above the eye (*Figure 6a*). In the older embryos, decapitation is required. The freed cerebral hemisphere can now be disconnected from the brain-stem by an incision across the pontine flexure (*Figure 6b* and *c*).

2. Lie brain so the surface of hemispheres faces you (*Figure 6d*).

3. Make incision close to midline along surface of each hemisphere with small iridectomy scissors (*Figure 6d* and *e*), making sure not to go too deep as this will damage striatal structures.

4. Splay open each hemisphere along cut surface, as the cut should lie along the complete anteroposterior axis of the lateral ventricles (*Figure 6e*).

5. On the lateral wall of each ventricle lies a bifid ridge of striatal tissue (*Figure 6f*).

6. Slice this ridge off with scissors by cutting adjacent to and parallel with the lateral wall of the venticle.

7. Repeat with the other hemisphere and then place striatal tissue into a separate dish of HBSS.

(c) Procedures for preparing, seeding, and culturing the striatal neurons are identical to those for nigral cells, i.e. *Protocols 4* and *5*.

(d) Characterization of GABAergic striatal neurons is performed using specific anti-GABA antibodies (see *Figure 7*). To reduce glial growth within the culture antimitotic agents can be added (see Introduction).

6. Concluding remarks

The culturing of nigral and striatal cells has gained prominence over recent years mainly as a result of the resurgence of interest in the neurodegenerative diseases of the CNS and the use of neural transplants as a possible treat-

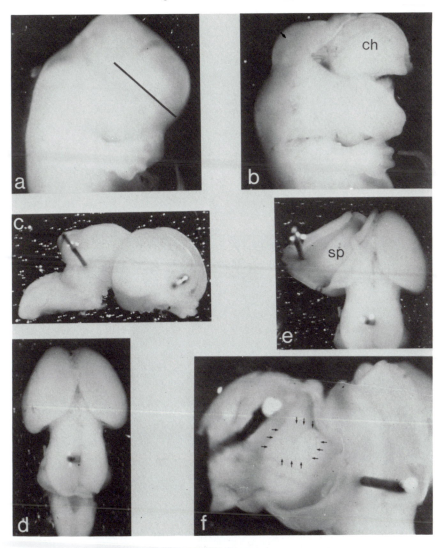

Figure 6. Dissecting out the striatal primordia. (a) After removal of the embryo and measuring its crl, an incision is made under the cerebral hemispheres just rostral to the eye. (b) The cerebral hemispheres (ch) emerge from beneath the skull and meninges and is removed by an incision at the level of the medulla/pons (→). (c) The brain including brain-stem is then removed and (d) placed so that the surface of the hemispheres is facing, and an incision is then made close to the midline in the anteroposterior direction. (e) The incision reveals the striatal primordia (sp). (f) The primordia consist of a bifid ridge which is removed by the undercutting of it (represented by the *arrows*).

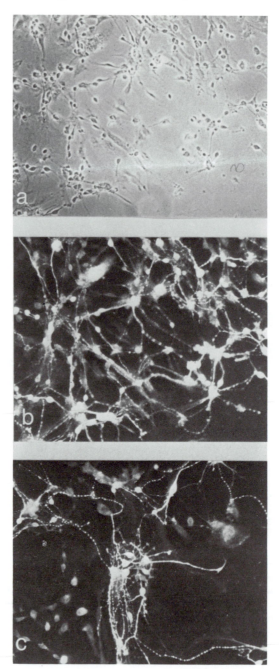

Figure 7. Cultured striatal neurons. (a) After three days in culture the neurons have developed large axonal arborizations. (b) The vast majority of these cells stain for GABA. (c) After eight days in the culture the fibre outgrowth has increased still further (× 200).

ment for them. The use of *in vitro* techniques enables the behaviour of cells to be investigated under clearly defined conditions, including their response to neurotoxic and neurotrophic factors. This has implications not only in terms of transplantation but also in terms of normal neural development and the aetiopathogenesis of these neurodegenerative diseases.

Acknowledgements

This work was largely supported by the MRC. We would like to thank Steve Dunnett, James Fawcett, Liz Housden, Roger Keynes, and Geoff Cook for their critical comments on the manuscript, and John Bashford for his help with the photography.

References

1. Forno, L. S. (1990). In *Parkinson's disease* (ed. G. Stern), pp. 185–238. Chapman and Hall, London.
2. Martin, J. P. and Gusella, J. F. (1986). *N. Engl. J. Med.*, **315**, 1267.
3. Dunnett, S. B. and Björklund, A. (1992). *Neural transplantation:a practical approach.* IRL Press, Oxford.
4. Prochiantz, A., Daquet, M.-C., Herbert, A., and Glowinski, J. (1979). *Proc. Natl. Acad. Sci. USA*, **76**, 5387.
5. Hemmendinger, L. M., Garber, B. B., Hoffmann, P. C., and Heller, A. (1981). *Proc. Natl. Acad. Sci. USA*, **78**, 1264.
6. Heyer, E. J. (1984). *Brain Res.*, **310**, 142.
7. AhnertHilger, G., Engele, J., Reisert, I., and Pilgrim, Ch. (1986). *Neuroscience*, **17**, 157.
8. Tomozawa, Y. and Appel, S. H. (1986). *Brain Res.*, **399**, 111.
9. Sanchez-Ramos, J., Barrett, J. N., Goldstein, M., Weiner, W. J., and Hefti, F. (1986). *Neurosci. Lett.*, **72**, 215.
10. Sanchez-Ramos, J., Michel, P., Weiner, W. J., and Hefti, F. (1988). *J. Neurochem.*, **50**, 1934.
11. Friedman, L. and Mytilineou, C. (1987). *Neurosci. Lett.*, **79**, 65.
12. Brundin, P., Barbin, G., Strecker, R. E., Isacson, O., Prochiantz, A., and Björklund, A. (1988). *Dev. Brain Res.*, **39**, 233.
13. Collier, T. J., Sladek, C. D., Gallagher, M. J., Blanchard, B. C., Daley, B. F., Foster, P. N., *et al.* (1988). *Prog. Brain Res.*, **78**, 631.
14. Dal Toso, R., Giorgi, O., Soranzo, C., Kirschner, G., Ferrari, G., Favaron, M., *et al.* (1988). *J. Neurosci.*, **8**, 733.
15. Ort, C. A., Futamachi, K. J., and Peacock, J. H. (1988). *Dev. Brain Res.*, **39**, 205.
16. Silva, N. A., Mariani, A. P., Harrison, N. L., and Barker, J. L. (1988). *Proc. Natl. Acad. Sci. USA*, **85**, 7346.
17. Ferrar, G., Minozzi, M.-C., Toffano, G., Leon, A., and Skaper, S. D. (1989). *Dev. Biol.*, **133**, 140.
18. Michel, P. P., Dandapani, B. K., Sanchez-Ramos, J., Efange, S., Pressman, B. C., and Hefti, F. (1989). *J. Pharmacol. Exp. Ther.*, **248**, 842.

19. Mount, H., Welnar, S., Quirion, R., and Boksa, P. (1989). *J. Neurochem.*, **52,** 1300.
20. Reisert, I., Engele, J., and Pilgrim, Ch. (1989). *Cell Tissue Res.*, **255,** 411.
21. Engele, J., Pilgrim, Ch., Kirsch, M., and Reisert, I. (1989). *Brain Res.*, **483,** 98.
22. Chabry, J., Checler, F., Vincent, J.-P., and Mazella, J. (1990). *J. Neurosci.*, **10,** 3916.
23. Cheng, C. H. K., Barnes, N. M., Costall, B., and Naylor, R. J. (1990). *Eur. J. Pharmacol.*, **183,** 2351.
24. Granneman, J. G. and Kapatos, G. (1990). *J. Neurochem.*, **54,** 1995.
25. Bijak, M., Jarolimek, W., and Misgeld, U. (1991). *Br. J. Pharmacol.*, **102,** 699.
26. Carvey, P. M., Ptak, L. R., Lo, E. R., Lin, D., Buhrfiend, C. M., Goetz, C. M., *et al.* (1991). *Exp. Neurol.*, **114,** 28.
27. Chalmers, R. M. E. and Fine, A. (1991). In *Intracerebral transplantation in movement disorders* (ed. O. Lindvall, A. Björklund, and H. Widner), pp. 333–42. Elsevier, Amsterdam.
28. Dana, C., Pelaprat, D., Vial, M., Brouard, A., Lhiaubet, A.-M., and Rostene, W. (1991). *Dev. Brain Res.*, **61,** 259.
29. Berger, B., Di Porzio, U., Daquet, M. C., Gay, M., Vigny, A., Glowinski, J., *et al.* (1982). *Neuroscience*, **7,** 193.
30. Driscoll, B. F., Law, M. J., and Crane, A. M. (1991). *J. Neurochem.*, **56,** 1201.
31. Engele, J. and Bohn, M. C. (1991). *J. Neurosci.*, **11,** 3070.
32. Grilli, M., Wright, A. G., and Hanbauer, I. (1991). *J. Neurochem.*, **56,** 2108.
33. Hama, T., Kushima, Y., Miyamot, M., Kubota, M., Takei, N., and Hatanaka, H. (1991). *Neuroscience*, **40,** 445.
34. Hyman, C., Hofer, M., Barde, Y.-A., Juhasz, M., Yancopoulos, G. D., Squinto, S. P., *et al.* (1991). *Nature*, **350,** 230.
35. O'Malley, E. K., Black, I. B., and Dreyfus, C. F. (1991). *Exp. Neurol.*, **112,** 40.
36. Brouard, A., Pelaprat, D., Dana, C., Vial, M., Lhiaubet, A.-M., and Rostene, W. (1992). *J. Neurosci.*, **12,** 1409.
37. Meyer, E., Fawcett, J. W., and Dunnett, S. B. (1993). *Dev. Brain Res.*, **72,** 253.
38. Panula, P., Rechardt, L., and Hervonen, H. (1979). *Neuroscience*, **4,** 235.
39. Panula, P., Rechardt, L., and Hervonen, H. (1979). *Neuroscience*, **4,** 1441.
40. Messer, A. (1977). *Brain Res.*, **130,** 1.
41. Messer, A. (1981). *Neuroscience*, **6,** 2677.
42. Barbin, G., Selak, I., and Manthorpe, M. (1984). *Neuroscience*, **12,** 33.
43. Weiss, S., Pin, J.-P., Sebben, M., Kemp, D. E., Sladeczek, F., Gabrion, J., *et al.* (1986). *Proc. Natl. Acad. Sci. USA*, **83,** 2238.
44. Kessler, J. A. (1986). *Dev. Biol.*, **113,** 77.
45. Murphy, S. N., Thayer, S. A., and Miller, R. J. (1987). *J. Neurosci.*, **7,** 4145.
46. Usanfi, K., Shingai, R., and Ban, T. (1987). *Brain Res.*, **420,** 167.
47. Surmeier, D. J., Kita, H., and Kitai, S. T. (1988). *Dev. Brain Res.*, **42,** 265.
48. Koh, J.-Y. and Choi, D. W. (1988). *Brain Res.*, **446,** 374.
49. Misgeld, U. and Dietzel, I. (1989). *Brain Res.*, **492,** 149.
50. Maus, M., Cordier, J., Glowinski, J., and Premont, J. (1989). *Eur. J. Neurosci.*, **1,** 154.
51. Freese, A., DiFiglia, M., Koroshetz, W. J., Beal, M. F., and Martin, J. B. (1990). *Brain Res.*, **521,** 254.
52. Mesco, E. R., Joseph, J. A., and Roth, G. S. (1992). *J. Neurosci. Res.*, **31,** 341.

4

Septal neurons

CLIVE SVENDSEN

1. Introduction

Interest in the septum stems from numerous studies showing that cholinergic neurons in this, and other regions of the basal forebrain appear to degenerate in Alzheimer's disease (AD). These express both low and high affinity receptors for nerve growth factor (NGF), and project to allo and neocortical regions which show pathological changes in AD. As *in vivo* studies have shown that NGF can reduce cholinergic cell death in the septum induced by axotomy of the rat fimbria/fornix (1), the prospect of using this factor to prevent these cells dying in AD has been suggested (2,3) and is now undergoing preliminary clinical trials.

In vitro models have been useful in determining the effects of growth factors on developing cholinergic basal forebrain neurons under conditions where the microenvironment of the cells can be easily manipulated. A range of trophic factors are known to support cultured septal cholinergic neurons with little or no effect on non-cholinergic neurons (4). Furthermore, cell death induced by NGF withdrawal can be prevented by protein synthesis inhibitors or by leaving the cultures to 'mature' *in vitro* suggesting that this model may be a good example of developmental cell death in a central population of neurons (5).

This chapter describes how septal neurons can be grown in culture for extended periods of time using a simple modification of the normal culture method used for septal cutures (6) which involves creating a limited diffusion layer above the cells by placing a coverslip on top of the culture. This method was previously shown to increase neuronal survival and decrease glial proliferation in hippocampal cultures by Brewer and Cotman (7). Using this method the effects of various factors on developmental cell death and cholinergic neuronal health can be assessed under controlled conditions.

Clive Svendsen

2. Standard techniques for culturing, staining, and counting septal neurons

2.1 The sandwich technique

The basic method for successfully culturing septal neurons with is given in *Protocols 1* and *2*. For more extensive details on determining the exact fetal age through palpation and removal of embryos please see Dunnett and Bjorklund (8) and Chapter 3 in this volume by Barker and Johnson. It is now well established that addition of NGF (20–100 ng/ml) at the time of plating can increase both the size and number of cholinergic neurons in these cultures. This trophic factor should be added if large numbers of cholinergic neurons are required.

Protocol 1. Removal of embryos and dissection of the septum

Equipment and reagents

- Hank's balanced salt solution (HBSS) without magnesium or calcium
- Barbiturate anaesthetic
- 100% alcohol
- A dissection microscope (for removal of brains and removal of septal tissue)
- Sterile plastic 10 cm diameter Petri dishes, 50 ml plastic tube

- Large scissors, large-toothed forceps, small scissors, medium serrated forceps, very fine Vannas spring iridectomy scissors (Fine Science Tools, Canada), two pairs of extra fine Dumont No. 5 forceps (all instruments should be sterilized by autoclaving or alcohol washing before use)

Method

1. Terminally anaesthetize pregnant rat (E16–17) using a lethal dose of barbiturate anaesthetic.

2. Sterilize the underbelly using 100% alcohol and open peritoneum to expose uterine horns.

3. Remove both uterine horns using sterile scissors and forceps and transfer to a 50 ml tube containing a small amount of HBSS.

4. Under sterile culture hood conditions transfer the embryos from the 50 ml tube to a 10 cm dish and carefully remove from the uterine sacs. Transfer each embryo to another 10 cm dish containing fresh HBSS. Measure the crown-rump length which should be between 17 and 19 mm (*Figure 1A*).

5. Decapitate all embryos and transfer heads to fresh HBSS.

6. Remove brain by gently inserting a pair of forceps under the developing cranium, teasing the tissue apart to expose the brain which can then be prised out using one of the forceps, and transferred to fresh HBSS in a 5 cm Petri dish.

7. With the dorsal surface of the brain facing upward (*Figure 1B*) carefully open the developing cortex by cutting along it's caudo/rostral length. This will expose the underlying striatal region (*Figure 1C*).

42

8. The septi are located rostrally either side of the midline and each has a distinctive ovoid shape (*Figure 1D*). Cut away the overlying midline cortex (*Figure 1D*) to expose both of the septi as shown in *Figure 1E*.

9. To remove the septal region cut behind it and pull the tissue forward and away from the rest of the brain. Separate the two septi by cutting between them and trim any attached menigial or cortical tissue (*Figure 1F*).

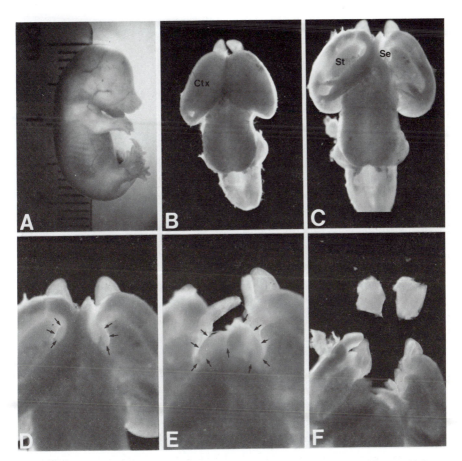

Figure 1. Dissection of the septum. (A) This shows the *maximum* size of fetus which can be used to successfully generate septal cultures. (B) Appearance of the isolated brain. (C) After removal of the overlying cortex (Ctx) the striatal eminance (St) and septum (Se) can be clearly distinguished. (D) High power view of the septum outlined by *arrows*. At this stage of the dissection there is still a layer of cortex over the medial aspect of the septum. (E) Following removal of the overlying cortex the whole septum is clearly seen and is outlined by *arrows*. (F) Carefully remove both septi and trim away any superfluous tissue.

Protocol 2. Preparation of tissue for plating

Equipment and reagents

- Final culture medium consisting of Dulbecco's modified eagles medium (DMEM, Imperial Labs) supplemented with 100 mM glutamine, 1 µl/ml antibiotic/antimitotic (Sigma), and 10% fetal calf serum (FCS, Imperial Labs): NGF (50 ng/ml) or other trophic factors can also be added to appropriate wells at this time
- 0.1% poly-L-lysine (Sigma) in sterile water
- 0.1% trypsin (Sigma) solution in sterile PBS
- 0.05% DNase solution (Sigma) in Hank's
- NUNC 24-well plates (obtainable from Gibco)
- 13 mm sterile glass coverslips (BDH)
- Sterile 10 ml and 5 ml pipettes, sterile glass pipettes
- Methanol lamp

Method

1. Add 300 µl of 0.1% poly-L-lysine to each well of a NUNC 24-well dish. Ensure even coverage of well surface and leave for 1 h before rinsing three times with sterile double distilled water. Add 1 ml of final culture medium and place in culture oven.

2. Transfer septal tissue pieces from 10–12 brains to 1 ml of 0.1% trypsin in a 10 ml centrifuge tube using a Pasteur pipette. Do not include too much HBSS which will dilute the trypsin (this can be avoided by allowing the septi to fall to the bottom of the pipette tip before transferring to the trypsin).

3. Leave in the trypsin for 20 min at 37 °C.

4. Carefully pour off the trypsin to waste leaving the septi at the bottom of the tube and then rinse in 10 ml of DMEM for 7 min.

5. Following two more 7 min rinses in DMEM add a final volume of 1.2–1.4 ml DMEM.

6. Using a fine-polished Pasteur pipette (to a tip diameter of about 0.45 mm), triturate the septi using the pipette until an even homogenate of cells is achieved (normally between 20 and 30 strokes are required).

7. Pipette 50 µl of the septal homogenate into each NUNC well prepared as described above (with 1 ml of serum-supplemented medium in each well). *It is crucial that once the septi are dissociated into suspension they are plated as soon as possible.* Any delay at this stage may result in severe clumping of the suspension. Although clumping following delay can be avoided by adding DNase more consistent results can be achieved by avoiding the use of such enzymes. This volume of suspension should result in a final plating density of approx. 100 000–150 000 cells/cm^2.

8. Transfer cells to the incubator and leave for 60 min.

9. Gently insert a sterile glass coverslip into each well so that it comes

to rest on top of the culture and the cells are 'sandwiched' between the coverslip and the bottom of the dish (see *Figure 2C*).

10. Five days following plating remove all serum-supplemented medium and replace with serum-free medium containing only added glutamine and antibiotics.

11. Change medium for new serum-free medium in all wells on a weekly basis.

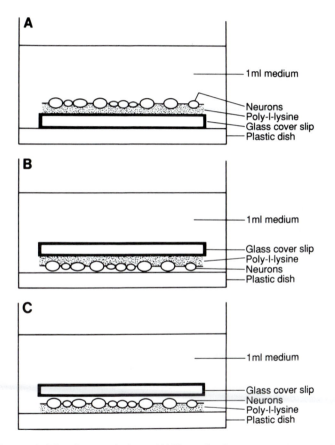

Figure 2. The sandwich culture technique. (A) Normal cultures are grown on glass coverslips coated with a suitable substrate and exposed to the medium above. (B) If the coverslip is turned upside-down (inverted) shortly after the cells have attached a sandwich condition is created where the cells are maintained in a small diffusion layer between the bottom of the well and the coverslip. (C) More consistent and even neuronal growth can be attained by coating the plastic bottom of the NUNC dish (plastic seems to combine with the substrate in a different way to glass) and dropping a non-coated coverslip on top shortly after plating.

3. Quantitative and qualitative analysis of septal cultures

3.1 Cell counting and area measurements

Cell counts can be performed on septal cultures grown in plastic NUNC dishes using either an inverted phase microscope with a camera lucida attachment, or an image analysis system. When counting either live or fixed cultures use x 16 objective to a project a 1 mm^2 field on to a sheet of paper via the camera lucida and mark the cells of interest (see next section for description of cell types). Count between four and six of these fields under blind conditions and average number of cells per field calculated for each culture dish. This number can then be multiplied by 100 to obtain the approximate density/cm^2 which is a convenient unit area measurement for cell density in most experiments. Area measurements or cell counts can also be made using standard image analysis techniques which are unique to the specific system purchased and cannot be detailed here.

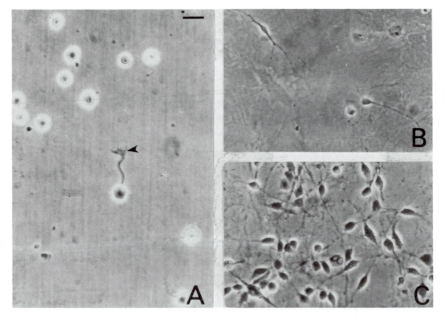

Figure 3. Appearance of septal cultures *in situ*. (A) A few hours after plating many phase-bright spheres can be seen, some of which are extending fine processes with growth cones (*arrow head*). (B) After 14 days *in vitro* using non-sandwich culture conditions many neurons have died and a monolayer of glia has developed. (C) In a sister well from the same culture grown using the sandwich technique there are significantly more neurons and no monolayer of glia (x 160).

3.2 Appearance of sandwich cultures and comparison with traditional methods

Two hours following plating septal cultures consist of many phase-bright spheres, some of which have begun to extend processes capped with growth cones (*Figure 3A*). If cultures are grown without using the sandwich method ('open faced' or normal culture conditions) you will find a significant amount of neuronal cell death and glial proliferation occurs over the first seven days *in vitro* (*Figure 3B*) when compared to sandwich cultures (*Figure 3C*) which can only be be attenuated by using higher plating densities (*Figure 4*).

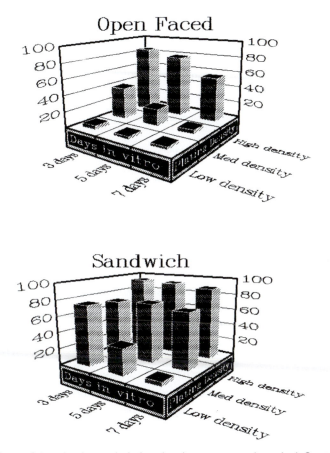

Figure 4. Effects of time *in vitro* and plating density on neuronal survival. Septal cultures were plated at high (200 000 cells/cm²), medium (100 000 cells/cm²), or low (25 000 cells/cm²) density. Note the significantly higher survival under all conditions for the septal cultures grown using the sandwich culture technique. Numbers expressed as percentage of neurons remaining (means from two representative experiments).

3.3 Staining methods to identify neurons and glia

Although the morphology of cells under phase-contrast may suggest either glial or neuonal phenotypes, confirmation is required using specific markers following fixation.

Protocol 3. Fixation and staining of septal cultures

Equipment and reagents

- 4% buffered paraformaldahyde (0.1 M) pH 7.4
- PBS or 0.1 M Tris buffer pH 7.4, 0.1 M sodium acetate buffer pH 6.0, 0.1 M sodium nitrate buffer pH 6.0
- Incubation medium for AChE staining: 50 mM acetate buffer pH 6.0 containing 5 mM sodium citrate, 3 mM cupric sulfate, 10 μM potassium ferricyanide, and 4 mM acetylthiocholine iodide substrate
- 0.1% silver nitrate solution in double distilled water
- Luxol fast blue solution (LFB): 0.1% in 70% alcohol
- Appropriate secondary biotin-conjugated secondary antiserum and ABC staining kit (Dako or Vector Labs, UK)
- Diaminobenzidine (DAB, 2 mg/ml) with H_2O_2 (5 μl/10 ml)

- Solid gelatine cubes (BDH)
- PBS or Tris buffer with azide (1 g/litre)
- Primary antibodies to glial fibrillary acidic protein (GFAP, 1 : 2700; Dako), neuron-specific enolase (NSE, 1 : 2000; Dako), microtubule associated protein 2 (MAP2, 1 : 1000, Sigma), choline acetyltransferase (ChAT, 1 : 12; from F. Eckenstein, Oregon Health Sciences University, Eugine, OR, USA), or low affinity NGF receptor (p75^{NGFR}, 1.5 μg/ml; from E. M. Johnson, Washington University, St. Louis, USA). These antibodies have been extensively used by the author on septal cultures and are known to work well. However, the same antiserum obtained from other commercial sources should also work but will need to be tested for efficacy at various concentrations.

A. Fixation

1. Prior to fixation, gently rotate the coverslips in the sandwich cultures within the culture dish in order to break the surface contact between the neurons and the glass before lifting. Without this step some neurons may be washed off due to the suction effect of raising the coverslip.

2. When the coverslip has been lifted using a pair of fine forceps with a hooked end, remove all of the culture medium and replace with 1 ml of 4% paraformaldehyde and leave for 25 min.

3. Wash wells three times with Tris buffer with azide.

B. Acetylcholinesterase histochemical staining for cholinergic neurons

1. Wash wells three times with sodium acetate buffer.

2. Add 1 ml of freshly made AChE incubation medium to each well.

3. After a 1 h incubation wash the wells in acetate buffer three times.

4. Add 1 ml of 2% ammonium sulfate for 1 min.

5. Wash again three times in *sodium nitrate* buffer.

6. Develop in silver nitrate solution for 1 min.

7. Wash well in sodium nitrate followed by acetate buffer.

---

8. Preserve cultures by removing the final rinse and adding five drops of heated (48 °C) liquid gelatine which then solidifies on cooling. If wells have been in the fridge allow them to warm to room temperature before adding the gelatine to avoid air bubble formation.

C. Immunocytochemical staining

1. Following 25 min fixation in 4% paraformaldehyde rinse wells three times with Tris buffer.

2. Add 1 ml of 1% goat serum and 0.2% Triton X in Tris buffer and leave for 1 h to block non-specific antigenic sites and permeate cell membranes. *Do not use Triton X when using antiserum to cell surface proteins such as the NGF receptor.*

3. Leave wells overnight at 4 °C in primary antibody made up with 1% goat serum in Tris buffer.

4. Following three 15 min washes in Tris with azide incubate for 1 h in the appropriate second antibody; anti-rat IgG for ChAT (1 : 40, Sigma), biotinylated anti-mouse IgG for p75[NGFR] and MAP2 (1 : 100, Sigma), and biotinylated anti-rabbit IgG for NSE and GFAP (1 : 100, Sigma).

5. Following another three washes in Tris buffer, cultures being stained for ChAT are then incubated for another hour in anti-rat PAP (1 : 40, Sera Labs). Cultures being stained for MAP2, GFAP, p75[NGFR], and NSE are incubated for 30 min in the ABC mix using the vecta staining kit (Vector Labs, UK).

6. Following three washes in Tris buffer add 1 ml of DAB solution for 5–10 min.

7. Wash three times in Tris buffer and mount in gelatine as described previously.

D. Cytological staining using LFB

This can be used as a counterstain for wells stained previously using immunocytochemical or histochemical methods.

1. Take cultures previously stained for AChE or non-stained cultures fixed for 25 min in 4% paraformaldehyde and rinse three times in Tris buffer.

2. Partially dehydrate in 50% alcohol for 30 min.

3. Remove alcohol and add 0.1% LFB in 70% alcohol for 1 h.

4. Rinse three times in double distilled water and mount in gelatine as described above.

The LFB stain was chosen from the many histological stains available as it was found to differentially stain neurons and astrocytes with the neurons hav-

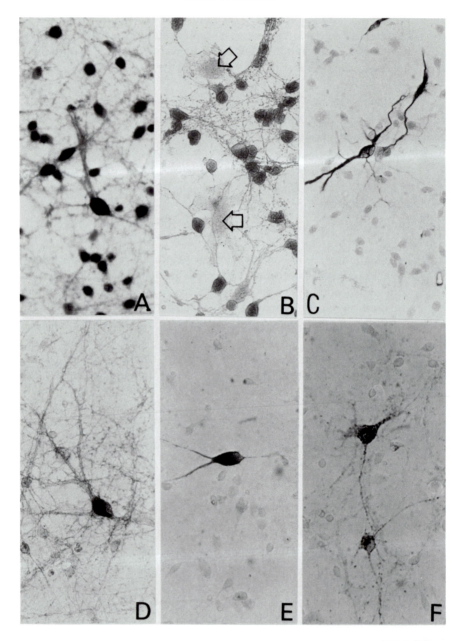

Figure 5. Septal cultures at 14 days *in vitro* stained for (A) LFB, (B) NSE where *arrows* represent unstained glia, (C) GFAP showing differentiated astrocytes, (D) AChE, (E) ChAT, and (F) P75^{NGFR} (x 250).

ing a characteristically dark stain and the astrocytes only staining very lightly (*Figure 5A*). Using NSE (a neuronal marker) and GFAP (a glial marker) immunocytochemistry, neurons and astrocytes can be more precisely identified in sandwich cultures where it is evident that there are many more neurons than astrocytes at 14 days *in vitro* (*Figure 5B*). Interestingly, the few glia present in sandwich cultures have a fibrous elongated structure (*Figure 5C*) which is very different to the squameous and rectangular shape of glia in normal open faced cultures.

After 14 days *in vitro,* staining for the various neuronal phenotypes can also be performed. When NGF is included in the medium at the time of plating, many AChE, ChAT, and P75[NGFR] positive neurons should be seen which are normally larger and fewer in number than other neurons in the culture. AChE and P75[NGFR] staining will label fibres and cell bodies whereas the ChAT staining will label the cell body and proximal dentrites only (*Figures 5D–F*). ChAT immunoulabelling is the most sensitive to changes in culture conditions (e.g. removal of trophic factor support) such that down-regulation of this enzyme will occur before there are visible alterations in staining for AChE or P75[NGFR] are detected. Under sandwich culture conditions septal cultures can be grown for five weeks without the formation of a glial monolayer (see Svendsen *et al.* 1994) and if NGF is present throughout this period the number of cholinergic neurons remains at a similar level, while the number of non-cholinergic neurons gradually decreases to approximately 10% of plating values by four weeks *in vitro* (*Table 1*). In older sandwich septal cultures (generally >18 days *in vitro*) you may find some cell death in the centre of the coverslip. In such cultures both non-cholinergic and cholinergic neurons can still be reliably counted in a 2 mm wide ring of growth towards the outside of the coverslip.

4. Variables that affect neuronal survival using the sandwich technique

The general outline of the development of septal cultures over time described in the previous sections is true for all cultures grown from E16–17

Table 1. Development of high density sandwich septal cultures with time *in vitro*

Time *in vitro*	Total neurons	Cholinergic neurons	Glia	Per cent Cholinergic
7 days	140 000	814	26 250	0.5
14 days	76 500	1136	19 375	1.4
21 days	60 200	928	16 250	1.5
28 days	22 500	784	12 500	3.4
35 days	15 625	992	15 600	6.0

All numbers expressed as cells/cm². Values represent means from duplicate wells in a typical experiment.

fetuses at an initial plating density of approximately 100 000 cells/cm² on poly-L-lysine coated plastic. When these three major variables are held constant (age of the fetuses, cell density, and substrate) you will find the sandwich technique to be remarkably consistent. However, certain small changes to these conditions have a profound effect on neuronal survival and are summarized below.

(a) Batches of serum *do* vary and although we found Imperial Labs to be the most most consistent supplier there may be the occasional batch which does not give consistent growth of the cultures. If there is not good neuronal survival using the sandwich technique try a new batch of serum either from the same company or another company.

(b) Growing septal cultures on inverted poly-L-lysine coated glass coverslips (see *Figure 1B*) gives similar results to growing them on plastic for the first week and has the benefit of being able to remove the coverslips and mount them on slides to be used with a regular microscope. However, septal cultures grown on glass coverslips were found to develop large regions of fasciculation and clumping between 7 and 14 days *in vitro*, particularly at low plating densities. Cultures grown on plastic very rarely showed this fasciculation effect and appeared to provide a better substrate for these cultures.

(c) If older fetuses are used to generate septal cultures there will be poorer long-term neuronal survival and increased numbers of glia using the sandwich culture method.

(d) If the final suspension is plated directly on to dry poly-L-lysine coated coverslip (rather than into 1 ml of medium) and the cells left to attach in this small volume for 10 min, approximately 30% of the cells lose their phase-brightness and degenerate within 3 h. However, this method has the advantage of only applying cells to a small region of the coverslip (but an adequate size for counting purposes) and even with the post-plating cell death results in an increased number of total cells per unit area. This technique may be useful when larger numbers of wells are required from a single experiment.

References

1. Williams, L. R., Varon, S., Peterson, G. M., Wictorin, K., Fischer, W., Bjorklund, A., *et al.* (1986). *Proc. Natl. Acad. Sci. USA*, **83,** 9231.
2. Hefti, F. (1983). *Ann. Neurol.*, **13,** 109.
3. Hefti, F., Hartikka, J., and Knusel, B. (1989). *Neurobiol. Aging*, **10,** 1.
4. Knusel, B., Michel, P. P., Schwaber, J. S., and Hefti, F. (1990). *J. Neurosci.*, **10,** 558.
5. Svendsen, C. N., Kew, J. N. C., Staley, K., and Sofroniew, M. V. (1994). *J. Neurosci.*, **14,** 75.

6. Hartikka, J. and Hefti, F. (1988). *J. Neurosci.*, **8,** 2967.
7. Brewer, G. J. and Cotman, C. W. (1989). *Brain Res.*, **494,** 65.
8. Dunnett, S. B. and Bjorklund, A. (1992). In *Neural transplantaion: a practical approach* (ed. S. B. Dunnet and A. Bjorklund), pp. 1–19. Oxford University Press, Oxford.

5

Proliferation and differentiation in retinal cell cultures

LAURA LILLIEN

1. Introduction

1.1 Retinal development *in vivo*

The vertebrate retina consists of seven major types of cells arranged in three layers that contain cell bodies, alternating with two layers that contain fibres and synapses (*Figure 1*). Different types of retinal cells can be distinguished by their morphology, expression of antigenic markers, and laminar position. For example, the cell bodies of rod and cone photoreceptor cells are found in the outer nuclear layer (ONL), bipolar, horizontal, amacrine, and Muller cells in the inner nuclear layer (INL), and ganglion cells in the layer closest to the vitreous. This complex structure develops from a small number of neuroepithelial cells that arise from an out-pocketing of the neural tube. During embryonic development, retinal progenitor cells divide extensively, and in some species, progenitor cells continue to divide during the postnatal period (1,2). Populations of progenitor cells that give rise to different types of retinal cells stop dividing at characteristic times during development, differentiate, and migrate to appropriate cell layers (2).

To find out more about the mechanisms that regulate the proliferation and differentiation of retinal cells, their clonal relationships were visualized by marking progenitor cells in the developing rodent retina (3–5). This was accomplished by introducing genes encoding enyzmes such as *E. coli* β-galactosidase or human placental alkaline phosphatase into retinal progenitor cells using retroviral vectors (3,5). The expression of these enzymes in individual cells could then be visualized by histochemical or immunohistochemical methods. The viruses used for these studies integrate stably into the DNA of the cells they infect, provided that the cells are still mitotic at the time of infection (6). The viruses used for studies of cell lineage were designed to be incapable of replicating to spread to neighbouring cells; therefore, the genes introduced via these vectors are passed on to the progeny of infected cells, but not to neighbouring cells, and the resulting clones of cells that express the

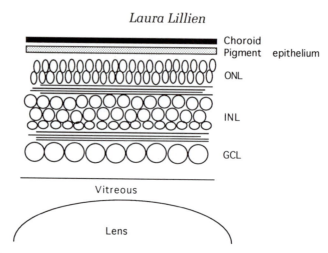

Figure 1. Schematic representation of a cross-section through the retina and surrounding ocular tissue showing three retinal layers that contain cell bodies (ONL: outer nuclear layer, INL: inner nuclear layer, GCL: ganglion cell layer) separated by layers of fibres and synapses (outer and inner plexiform layers). Compare to *Figure 4*.

marker can be analysed when development has been completed. In this way it is possible to determine the number and types of cells that individual progenitor cells give rise to, as a measure of proliferation and differentiation, respectively. Using this technique, clones containing multiple types of retinal cells were observed, and the number of cells in a clone was shown to vary over a wide range (3–5). The results of these studies indicated that most retinal cells were not rigidly restricted at early stages of development in their capacity to divide or to develop into particular types of cells. This suggested that extracellular signals play an important role in regulating the proliferation and diversification of retinal progenitor cells (3,4). In order to facilitate the identification of these signals, and the mechanisms that regulate competence to respond to them, several laboratories have developed a number of *in vitro* systems which allow manipulations of cells and signals that are much more difficult to perform *in vivo*. Most of the examples given in this chapter refer to rodent cells, though similar manipulations and strategies can be applied to retinal cells from other sources.

1.2 Use of *in vitro* systems to study the control of retinal development

Several kinds of *in vitro* preparations are available for studying retinal development. In one type of *in vitro* system, cell–cell signalling is disrupted by physically separating cells from each other. These dissociated cells can be cultured at different cell densities to determine whether processes of interest depend on cell–cell interactions (7,8). For example, if a process such as the development of cell type 'X' does not occur at low cell densities, but does occur at higher cell densities, this suggests that signals from other types of cells are involved in the development of cell type 'X'. The low density cultures, referred to below as 'minimal' culture preparations, can then be used to test candidate signals, for example, to determine whether they can restore the development of cell type 'X' (7,8). In other kinds of culture preparations, endogenous signalling among cells is optimized, and many processes approximate development *in vivo*. These 'maximal' preparations include explants (9), slices (10), and cell aggregates (11–14). Candidate signals can be added to 'maximal' preparations to determine whether excess levels of a signal can alter proliferation, bias the choice of cell type, or disrupt retinal histogenesis; alternatively, neutralizing antibodies can be added to determine whether they can inhibit any of these processes, to demonstrate the physiological function of the endogenous signal.

2. Culture preparation

2.1 Culture media

For most applications, culture medium containing defined supplements is used rather than serum, because components in serum may mimic/mask effects of the signals to be tested. For normal retinal histogenesis to occur, however, serum-containing medium is used, because lamination does not develop as well in the absence of serum.

2.1.1 Serum-free medium

(a) 50% Dulbecco's modified Eagle medium (DMEM; Gibco-BRL) containing D-glucose (4500 mg/ml) and sodium pyruvate (110 mg/ml), but no L-glutamine, and 50% Ham's F-12 nutrient mixture (Gibco-BRL), preferably without L-glutamine.

(b) Penicillin–streptomycin at 500 U/ml each (Gibco-BRL), added from a 100 x stock (stored –20 °C).

(c) Modified N2 supplement (13), added from a 10 × stock (*Table 1*; all components available from Sigma), or 100 x stock (from Gibco-BRL). Stocks stored –20 °C. If 10 x stock is prepared, the 1 x medium should be filtered to sterilize (0.2 μm filter, Gelman or Millipore, low protein binding); the 100 x stock from Gibco-BRL is already sterile.

(d) Bovine insulin (Sigma, I 6634), 5 μg/ml final concentration, added from a 100 x stock, made up in 0.1 M HCl and passed through a 0.2 μm low protein binding filter. Insulin stocks should be stored at 4 °C, for no longer than six weeks.

2.1.2 Serum-containing medium

This is made up in 50% DMEM/50% Ham's F-12 containing 500 U of penicillin–streptomycin. Instead of, or in addition to, the components in the

Table 1. Composition of modified N2 supplement for serum-free cultures

	Final concentration (1x)
Human transferrin	100 µg/ml
BSA (fatty acid-free, fraction V)	100 µg/ml
Putrescine	16 µg/ml
Progesterone	62.5 ng/ml
Selenium	40 ng/ml
Thyroxine	40 ng/ml
Triiodothyronine	3.35 ng/ml

modified N2 supplement, 5% fetal bovine serum (FBS) is used. Others have used 10% FBS or 5% rat serum and rat embryo extract and have obtained similar results (9,11).

2.2 Dissection of retina

For rat retinal cultures, best results are obtained using retinal tissue from embryonic day 14 to new-born stages. Dissection of younger tissue is more difficult, while the survival of cells from older retinas may present problems and require the addition of survival factors. For some applications, it may be preferable to minimize the number of non-retinal cells, such as astrocytes and endothelial cells, in the cultures. These cells are associated with the vasculature, and populate the retina beginning in the central region, spreading to the periphery as development proceeds (15). Their numbers can therefore be reduced by using only the peripheral part of the retina when preparing the cultures (7).

Protocol 1. Dissection of retinal tissue

Equipment and reagents
- Hank's balanced salt solution (HBSS, Gibco-BRL), 4 °C or room temperature
- Sterile No. 5 forceps (two or three pairs), and iridectomy scissors
- Sterile 35 mm or 60 mm plastic Petri or tissue culture dishes

Method

1. Remove eyes and place in dish containing HBSS, on ice or at room temperature.

2. Using two forceps, carefully remove choroidal and pigment epithelial membranes to reveal retina, and cut off optic nerve if still attached (as shown in *Figure 2a*). Gently separate retina from lens and vitreous (*Figure 2b*), and transfer retina to another dish containing HBSS using a wide-bore pipette. Pool retinas from 2–20 eyes.

3. If all of the retina is to be used, cut into small pieces, approx. 0.5–1.0 mm². If only peripheral retina is to be used, cut off a strip around the periphery approx. 1–2 mm wide (*Figure 2c*), and then cut this strip into small pieces.

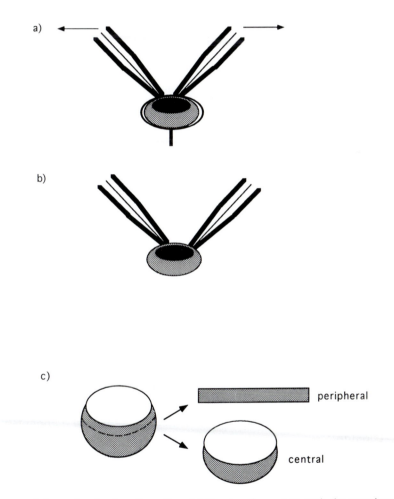

a)

b)

c)

peripheral

central

Figure 2. Schematic of retina dissection. (a) Use two forceps to grab the membranes at the anterior surface of the dissected eye and pull apart to separate the retina and lens (grey and black) from the scleral, choriodal, and pigment epithelial membranes that surround the retina (thick black line). The optic nerve (at the posterior part of the eye) can be cut off if still attached. (b) Use two forceps to separate the retina (grey) from the lens (black). (c) The retina can be separated into central and peripheral regions by cutting away a peripheral strip using iridectomy scissors.

2.3 'Minimal' systems: monolayer and collagen gel cultures

2.3.1 Tissue dissociation

Retinal cells can be separated from each other using mechanical or enzymatic methods (9,12,16,19). A procedure using trypsin is given in *Protocol 2*, though others have also used papain to dissociate retinal cells (17).

Protocol 2. Dissociation of retinal cells

Equipment and reagents
- Sterile 15 ml polystyrene centrifuge tubes
- 0.1% trypsin (Type III, Sigma, T8253) in Ca^{2+}/Mg^{2+}-free HBSS (from 10 x stock stored at –20 °C), warmed to room temperature before adding to retinal tissue
- Water-bath at 37 °C
- Centrifuge (for example, IEC bench-top with swinging bucket rotor)
- 0.4 mg/ml trypsin inhibitor (soybean or egg white, Sigma, T2011), plus 0.4 mg/ml DNase I (Type IV, Sigma, D5025) in DMEM (filtered and stored in 1–2 ml aliquots at –20 °C): warm to room temperature before adding to retinal tissue
- Complete culture medium, with or without serum, at 37 °C

Method

1. After dissecting retina and cutting into small pieces, transfer pieces to centrifuge tube using Pasteur pipette, and remove excess HBSS.

2. Rinse pieces of retina with approx. 0.5 ml of trypsin solution (add and remove immediately).

3. Add approx. 1 ml of trypsin solution to the centrifuge tube. Incubate pieces of retina in trypsin at 37 °C for 20–30 min (time depends on age: less time may be needed for younger tissue).

4. Add 0.5 ml of trypsin inhibitor plus DNase solution and 0.5 ml of culture medium to tube. Triturate (pipette up and down five to ten times) gently with a Pasteur pipette to separate pieces into single cells. If pieces remain, let them settle to the bottom of the tube (2–3 min), and carefully remove medium above them containing single cells. Trituration of the residual pieces can be repeated, and the suspensions containing single cells pooled.

5. Pellet cells by centrifugation for 3–5 min at approx. 400 *g*, room temperature.

6. Aspirate supernatant, resuspend cells in small volume of medium (100–500 µl), and count 100 × dilution using haemocytometer.

2.3.2 Monolayer cultures

After retinal cells have been dissociated, they can be diluted in culture medium and plated at different cell densities on plastic tissue culture dishes or glass coverslips (cleaned with 100% ethanol, rinsed with tissue culture grade water, and baked to sterilize) coated with a variety of substrates (see

Introduction, Chapter 1). Cells plated at densities of 25 000 or more cells per 12 cm coverslip should survive well for at least three days *in vitro* without additional survival factors (7). For longer periods of culture, addition of survival factors may be necessary, or higher cell densities can be used (7). If cultures are maintained for more than three days *in vitro*, approximately half of the medium should be replaced with fresh culture medium every three to four days. For some applications, i.e. very low cell densities, survival can be improved by using feeder layers of irradiated cells such as CNS astrocytes (see Chapter 7). When cells for feeder layers become confluent, proliferation can be arrested by exposure to an X-ray source (2700 rads). Dissociated retinal cells can then be placed on top of the monolayer of irradiated feeder cells.

2.3.3 Gel cultures

While cells plated as monolayers start out well separated from each other, over several days *in vitro* they tend to form small clusters and grow processes that may contact other cells. To reduce cell–cell interactions to a greater extent, dissociated cells can be cultured in a support matrix of collagen (type 1, bovine skin, Collaborative Research) (8). To form the gel, dissociated cells (e.g. 5×10^5–2×10^7 cells/ml) are mixed with 1.2 mg/ml collagen plus 100 mM Hepes (pH 7.3) in culture medium. After 30 min at 37 °C, gels are covered with culture medium. In addition to maintaining better cell separation, the use of a three-dimensional matrix may be important for the development of some types of retinal cells, such as rod photoreceptors (8).

2.4 'Maximal' systems: aggregate and explant cultures

Aggregate cultures can be made in two ways: by slow re-aggregation of dissociated cells, using rotation (12,14), or by rapid re-aggregation, using centrifugation to form a cell pellet (11). When cells are re-aggregated slowly, they can 'sort out', depending on the relative expression of adhesion molecules on different cells (18). By contrast, when cells are re-aggregated rapidly, they remain more randomly mixed, which is preferable for applications such as 'transplantation' *in vitro* (see below) (11).

Protocol 3. Re-aggregate cultures

1. For rapid re-aggregation, cells (e.g. 150 000–200 000 cells in 0.5 ml of medium) are centrifuged at 400 *g* for 7 min and left in the centrifuge tubes for 1 h at room temperature (11).

2. Pellets of cells are dislodged from the bottoms of the tubes by gently pipetting against the pellet with a Pasteur pipette. Even if cultures are to be maintained in serum-free medium, it is preferable to form pellets in medium that contains FBS, because pellets formed in the

---

Protocol 3. *Continued*

absence of serum have a greater tendency to break up when dislodged from the centrifuge tubes.

3. Using a Pateur pipette, pellets are transferred to the tops of nucleopore filters (13 mm diameter, 0.2 μm pore size, Costar) floating in 1.5 ml of culture medium in 35 mm tissue culture dishes (*Figure 3*).

4. Filters are prepared by boiling for 5 min in tissue culture grade water. When water has cooled, filters are transferred to sterile plastic Petri dishes with forceps. Filters have a shiny side and a dull side. When dried, filters are transferred to 35 mm dishes containing 1.5 ml of medium, and placed shiny side down, i.e. tissue is placed on the dull side.

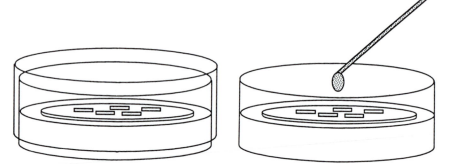

Figure 3. Schematic representation of explants or cell pellets supported on nucleopore filters floating in 35 mm tissue culture dishes.

Protocol 4. Explant cultures

1. When retinas are dissected from 13–15 day embryos, they may be left attached to vitreal and lens tissue after removal of choroidal and pigment epithelial membranes (9); alternatively, after removal of vitreal and lens tissue, retinas at any age may be left intact, or cut into small pieces as described in *Protocol 1*. This tissue can be transferred, using a Pasteur or wide-bore pipette, to the tops of nucleopore filters floating in 1.5 ml of medium in 35 mm tissue culture dishes as described above (*Figure 3*).

2. Alternatively, retinas can be allowed to attach to the bottoms of culture dishes coated with laminin, fibronectin, or dried films of rat tail collagen (9). Attachment is facilitated by using a small volume of medium when explants are initially placed on the culture surface. More medium is then added 3 h later. Methocel (0.7%, Dow Chemical)

can be used to increase the viscosity of the medium and reduce the likelihood of detachment (9). When cultured in the presence of serum, retinal explants develop cell and fibre layers as observed *in vivo* (*Figure 4*) (9). Distinct layers do not form as well if explants are cultured without serum.

3. Explants can be maintained for several weeks, replacing 0.5 ml of culture medium every three to four days. Agents to be tested on explants, such as growth factors and antibodies, should be added to the culture medium in the dish, and 30–50 µl of the diluted agent in culture medium can then be added to the tops of the filters supporting retinal explants (*Figure 3*).

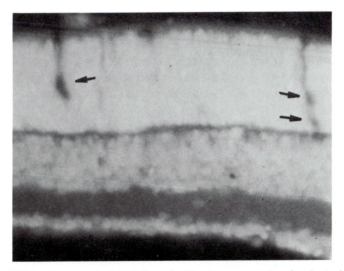

Figure 4. Section of retinal explant infected with virus expressing β-galactosidase and stained with DAPI to reveal lamination. New-born retinal explants were infected and cultured for one week on nucleopore filters. They were fixed in 0.5% glutaraidehyde, processed for X-Gal histochemistry, embedded in gelatine, frozen, sectioned (30 µm), and stained with DAPI. Most of the infected cells (*arrows*) develop into rod photoreceptors, located in the outer nuclear layer, as expected at this stage of development.

3. Use of retroviruses expressing lineage markers

Dividing retinal cells can be labelled by infecting *in vitro* at the time that cells are placed in culture by adding virus that expresses a lineage marker such as β-galactosidase to the culture medium (for example, 100–100 000 c.f.u. in 1–10 µl/culture). Detailed methods describing the preparation, storage, and use of viral stocks have been described elsewhere (6). For explants, infection is most efficient if virus is added (in a volume of 10–30 µl) after explants are placed on nucleopore filters floating in 1.5 ml of medium (*Figure 3*). The virus solution should contain 10% FBS, though it is not necessary to use polybrene to obtain high frequencies of infection. After several days or weeks, the expression of β-galactosidase in retinal cells can be visualized histochemically or immunohistochemically. Several commercial sources of antibodies are available. Detailed methods for histochemical detection have been described elsewhere (3,4,6). In both explant and monolayer cultures, cells in a clone tend to remain clustered (3–5); the number of cells in clones can be counted as a measure of the proliferation that has occurred during the interval following infection. Virus expressing alkaline phosphatase (AP) can also be used (5), but because AP is located on cell surfaces, and clones of labelled cells tend to form tight clusters, it is more difficult to distinguish individual cells and count them, compared to infection with virus expressing β-galactosidase.

4. Differentiation

Cell type in either 'minimal' or 'maximal' culture preparations can be identified using immunocytochemical markers. In preparations in which histogenesis occurs, such as explants, the laminar position and morphology of infected cells can also be used to assign cell type.

4.1 Cell type markers

A number of immunocytochemical markers for retinal cells have been described (20). Some of these antibodies label most of the cells in a class, such as rod photoreceptors or ganglion cells, while others may label more than one class of cells, or subpopulations of a class of cells. A list of some of the markers described for rodent retinal cells, with some information about labelling specificity *in vivo* and *in vitro*, is shown in *Table 2*. Many types of retinal cells can develop from dividing progenitor cells in 'minimal' culture systems. These include amacrine, bipolar, Muller, and ganglion cells (7,8,19,21). Rod photoreceptor development is facilitated by using collagen gels (8), or substrates containing S-laminin (22), compared to monolayer cultures on other substrates such as poly-D-lysine, laminin, or collagen (7–9,11).

4.2 Lineage markers

In explant cultures grown in serum, cell and fibre layers develop as observed *in vivo* (see below) (9). If explants are infected with a virus that expresses the lineage marker β-galactosidase, the fate of cells that are mitotic at the time of infection can be determined after several days or weeks by examination of the morphology and laminar position of the labelled cells following histochemical staining and sectioning. An example of labelled cells in a cross-section of an infected retinal explant is shown in *Figure 4*. The identity of the infected cells can be confirmed by double label immunocytochemistry, using

Table 2. Antibodies that label retinal cells

Antibody (antigen)	Labelling specificity
Ret P1 (rhodopsin)	Rod photoreceptors (26)
115A10 (surface)	Bipolar cells (27)
L7	Bipolar cell (28)
HPC-1 (syntaxin)	Amacrine cells (19)
Neurofilament	Horizontal and ganglion cells (29)
TUJ-1 (tubulin)	Ganglion cells (30)
Ret-G2	Muller glial cells (26)
Tyrosine hydroxylase	Subpopulation of amacrine cells (31)

antibodies to β-galactosidase in combination with cell type antibodies, such as those listed in *Table 2*. In this way, lineage studies can be extended to a more accessible system; for example, the effects of altering the environment on cell lineage can be determined by adding growth factors or neutralizing antibodies to explants infected with a virus that expresses a lineage marker. Moreover, viruses can be used to introduce bioactive genes or antisense sequences in combination with lineage markers to determine whether mis-expression of normal or mutated forms of the genes can perturb development (23).

4.3 Lamination

In vivo, the three layers that contain the cell bodies of retinal neurons, glial cells, and photoreceptor cells become discernible by the end of the first post-natal week in the rodent retina. These layers can be visualized easily by staining with dyes such as DAPI (Molecular Probes) which bind to DNA. If retinal explants are grown in medium that contains serum, similar layers of cell bodies alternating with layers of fibres and synapses can be seen in sections of explants stained with DAPI (*Figure 4*). The presence of appropriate types of cells in the DAPI-labelled layers can be confirmed in sections stained with some of the antibodies listed in *Table 2*, and the presence of synapse-associated antigens in the DAPI-negative layers can be confirmed by staining with antibodies to synaptophysin, which labels synaptic vesicles (9). Although explants of new-born retina have cells in the layer appropriate for ganglion cells after one week *in vitro*, these do not appear to be ganglion cells. The survival of ganglion cells in explants can be enhanced by growth factors or conditioned medium (24).

4.4 'Transplantation' *in vitro*

The temporal patterns of proliferation and differentiation that have been observed in the retina *in vivo* have led to the suggestion that the extracellular signals that influence these processes may change during development, and/or the competence of progenitor cells to respond to such signals may change. One way to address the contributions of these mechanisms to retinal development is to expose retinal progenitor cells to different aged environments, for example, by mixing a small number of E15 cells with an excess of new-born cells, or vice versa, and asking whether the proliferation and/or differentiation of the small population of cells is altered by the large population of cells from a different developmental stage (11). To do this, it is necessary to mark the small population of cells in a way that will allow them to be distinguished days or weeks later from the excess of unmarked cells taken from retinas at other stages of development. Cells can be marked by exposing them to bromodeoxyuridine (11) or virus that expresses a lineage marker, prior to dissociation and mixing with cells from other stages of development. Alternatively, tissue from transgenic mice that express a marker such as β-galactosidase in retinal cells can be mixed with cells from mice that do not express this marker (25). The proliferation and differentiation of the marked populations of cells can then be analysed. When these manipulations were performed by Watanabe and Raff using E15 and P1 retinal cells, they observed that the proliferation of E15 cells was not altered by the older environment (excess unmarked P1 cells), nor was the proliferation of P1 cells altered by the younger environment (11). The development of P1 cells into rod photoreceptors was delayed by the younger cells, however, and the development of the E15 cells into rods was enhanced by the older environment, but could not be induced prematurely (11). These observations support the hypothesis that retinal progenitor cells change during development.

References

1. Denham, S. (1967). *J. Embryol. Exp. Morphol.*, **18**, 53.
2. Young, R. W. (1985). *Anat Rec.*, **212**, 199.
3. Turner, D. L. and Cepko, C. L. (1987). *Nature*, **328**, 131.
4. Turner, D. L., Snyder, E. Y., and Cepko, C. L. (1990). *Neuron*, **4**, 833.
5. Fields-Barry, S. C., Halliday, A. L., and Cepko, C. L. (1992). *Proc. Natl. Acad. Sci. USA*, **89**, 693.
6. Price, J., Turner, D., and Cepko, C. L. (1987). *Proc. Natl. Acad. Sci. USA*, **84**, 156.
7. Lillien, L. and Cepko, C. (1992). *Development*, **115**, 253.
8. Altshuler, D. and Cepko, C. L. (1992). *Development*, **114**, 947.
9. Sparrow, J. R., Hicks, D., and Barnstable, C. J. (1990). *Dev. Brain Res.*, **51**, 69.
10. Mack, A. F. and Fernald, R. D. (1992). *Exp. Neurol.*, **115**, 65.
11. Watanabe, T. and Raff, M. C. (1990). *Neuron*, **4**, 461.
12. Akagawa, K., Hicks, D., and Barnstable, C. J. (1987). *Brain Res.*, **437**, 298.
13. Bottenstein, J. E. and Sato, G. H. (1979). *Proc. Natl. Acad. Sci. USA*, **76**, 514.
14. Vollmer, G. and Layer, P. G. (1986). *J. Neurosci.*, **6**, 1885.
15. Stone, J. and Dreher, Z. (1987). *J. Comp. Neurol.*, **255**, 35.
16. Akagawa, K. and Barnstable, C. J. (1986). *Brain Res.*, **383**, 110.
17. Heuttner, J. E. and Baughman, R. W. (1986). *J. Neurosci.*, **6**, 3044.

18. Sheffield, J. B. and Moscona, A. A. (1970). *Dev. Biol.*, **23,** 36.
19. Anchan, R. M., Reh, T. A., Angello, J., Balliet, A., and Walker, M. (1991). *Neuron*, **6,** 923.
20. Barnstable, C. J. (1987). *Immunol. Rev.*, **100,** 47.
21. Reh, T. A. and Kljavin, I. J. (1989). *J. Neurosci.*, **9,** 4179.
22. Hunter, D. D., Murphy, M. D., Olsson, C. V., and Brunken, W. J. (1992). *Neuron*, **8,** 399.
23. Ghattas, I. R., Sanes, J. R., and Majors, J. E. (1991). *Mol. Cell. Biol.*, **11,** 5848.
24. de Araujo, E. G. and Linden, R. (1990). *Braz. J. Med. Biol. Res.*, **23,** 743.
25. Friedrich, G. and Soriano, P. (1991). *Genes Dev.*, **5,** 1513.
26. Barnstable, C. J. (1980). *Nature*, **286,** 231.
27. Onoda, N. and Fujita, S. C. (1987). *Brain Res.*, **416,** 359.
28. Oberdick, J., Smeyne, R. J., Mann, J. R., Zackson, S., and Morgan, J. I. (1990). *Science*, **248,** 223.
29. Barnstable, C. J., Hofstein, R., and Akagawa, K. (1985). *Dev. Brain Res.*, **20,** 286.
30. Lee, M. K., Tuttle, J. B., Rebhun, L. I., Cleveland, D. W., and Frankfurter, A. (1990). *Cell Motil. Cytoskel.*, **17,** 118.
31. Wulle, I. and Schnitzer, J. (1989). *Dev. Brain Res.*, **48,** 59.

6

Purified embryonic motoneurons

CHRISTOPHER E. HENDERSON, EVELYNE BLOCH-GALLEGO,
and WILLIAM CAMU

1. Introduction

Spinal motoneurons have been the object of much study using *in vivo* models, but their detailed study *in vitro* has been hindered by the cellular complexity of the spinal cord and the consequent difficulties in reproducibly obtaining pure motoneurons in culture. Since the 1970s different methods have been developed for their enrichment, identification, and/or purification. These methods are based on three major properties of the motoneuron: its localization in the ventral spinal cord, its relatively large size, and the fact that its axon projects to the limb bud from early stages (for a more complete review, see ref. 1). Each method has its special advantages and drawbacks: in general, those methods that give a high degree of purification have relatively low yields. Depending on the experiments to be performed, one method may be preferred to another.

In this article, we present the two techniques that we have found to be most useful on a day to day basis (*Figure 1*). The combination of the two techniques provides preparations that are consistently greater than 90% pure, sufficient for virtually every experimental need. The first technique, metrizamide density gradient centrifugation, was first developed by Schnaar and Schaffner (2) to enrich for large, buoyant cells and has since been modified by others, including ourselves (3–5). The second approach, immunopanning using antibodies to specific motoneuron cell surface antigens, has been developed in our laboratory for chicken and rat motoneurons (1,5–7). The antigen used for chicken motoneurons is that recognized by the SC1 and BEN monoclonal antibodies, a cell surface protein belonging to the immunoglobulin superfamily. Within the embryonic chicken spinal cord, it is expressed only by motoneurons and floor-plate (8) (*Table 1*). For rat motoneurons, we have used the Ig-192 antibody to the p75 low affinity neurotrophin receptor, which is expressed selectively by motoneurons within the ventral spinal cord from E14 onwards (9) (*Table 1*).

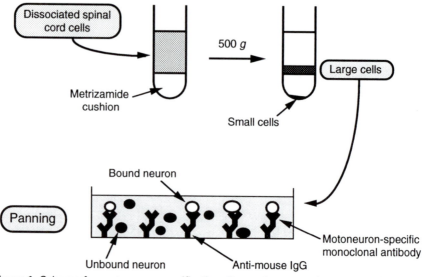

Figure 1. Scheme for motoneuron purification. Depending on embryo age and species (see text), the metrizamide and immunopanning steps may be used singly or, as here, sequentially for a high degree of purification.

2. Purification strategy

The protocols contained in this chapter are mostly self-explanatory and are therefore presented sequentially, without further introduction. However, before setting out to purify motoneurons, it is useful to consider which preparation is the most appropriate for a given experimental need.

2.1 Choice of species

Chicken embryos are easy and inexpensive to obtain. The purification of chick motoneurons and their culture are undoubtedly easier than for rat motoneurons. However, they do not respond in culture to factors such as the neurotrophins (4,5), and may be inappropriate for use with some antibodies. Rat motoneuron purification works reproducibly in our hands, but the cells are less robust. However, they are large and develop fast in culture. Mouse motoneurons are not currently accessible using immunopanning as there is no specific antibody to a cell surface antigen, but can in principle be enriched using metrizamide gradients at early stages.

2.2 Choice of embryo age

The methods described here may in practice be used for chicken embryos between E4 and E7, and for rat embryos between E14 and E15. The limiting factors are varied: the difficulty of gently dissociating older spinal cords, the

Table 1. Reagents required for motoneuron purification

Product	Source	Solution	Aliquots	Store at:	Comments
Anti-mouse Ig	Cappel, 55482	2 mg/ml	—	4 °C	Very stable
BSA	Sigma, A3311	4% (w/v) in L-15	10 ml	4 °C	Dialyse against L-15 if toxic
DNase I	Sigma, DN-25	1 mg/ml in L-15	500 µl	−20 °C	—
Glucose	Any	72 mg/ml in L-15	5 ml	−20 °C	—
Horse serum	Any	—	10 ml	−20 °C	Test batches before ordering
L-15 medium	Any	—	500 ml	4 °C	Test batches; extra cost of liquid medium is worth it
Laminin	Gibco-BRL, or home-made	1.5 mg/ml in PBS (500 ×)	1 ml	−70 °C	Always thaw on ice to prevent gelling, then keep at 4 °C
Metrizamide	Serva	6.5% or 6.8% in L-15	10 ml	4 °C	Store in full, capped tubes
Monoclonal antibodies	Hybridomas may now be obtained, with permission, from several laboratories	Saturated culture supernatant	10 ml	−20 °C	Commercially available 192 antibody (Boehringer) is effective but costly
Muscle extract	Prepare from neonatal chick muscle[a]	5 mg/ml	20 µl	−70 °C	Spin in micro-centrifuge after thawing
Neurotrophins	Genentech, Regeneron, Amgen	1 µg/ml in PBS, with 10% serum	50 µl	−70 °C	Stable for weeks at 4 °C
Penicillin–streptomycin	Any	10 000 U/ml–10 µg/ml (100 ×)	100 µl	−20 °C	—
Poly-D,L-ornithine	Sigma, P8638	1.5 mg/ml in in water (1000 ×)	20 µl	−20 °C	Other molecular weights also work
Sodium bicarbonate	Any	7.5% (w/v) water	—	+20 °C	—
Trypsin	Gibco-BRL	2.5% (w/v)	50 µl	−20 °C	

—[a] Protocol in ref. 7.

non-specific expression of the antigen used for panning at earlier stages, etc. The methods may undoubtedly be adapted for other stages if required, but this will require careful optimization and controls for specificity.

2.3 Choice of purification method

This is a function of the species and age of embryo being used and of the experimental needs, both quantitative and qualitative. Metrizamide centrifu-

Protocol 1. *Continued*

2. Transfer to a silicone support under a dissecting microscope. Remove head, tail, and bulk of viscera using forceps as scissors.

3. Use one pair of forceps to stabilize the embryo in the dish. Insert one point of the other pair into the central canal of the rostral spinal cord. Close forceps and use as scissors to tear dorsal tissue away over a distance of about 2 mm. Repeat this operation so as to open the spinal cord dorsally over the whole rostro-caudal extent of the embryo (*Figure 2A*).

4. Insert one pair of closed forceps between the dorsal lip of the spinal cord and the surrounding tissue at a point approximately opposite the forelimb bud. Slide the forceps rostrally and then caudally along the line of lowest resistance. Turn the embryo and repeat the operation on the other side; the cord should be well separated, although with rat embryos some meninges and dorsal root ganglia remain attached (*Figure 2B*).

5. If necessary, perform dorso-ventral dissection of **chicken** spinal cord at this stage. Use microscissors to trim simultaneously both dorsal lips of the cord still held in the embryo.

6. After freeing the ventral face of the spinal cord from the embryo (*Figure 2C*), remove the whole cord. If necessary, hold the rostral end of the cord with forceps and pull the meninges away in a rostro-caudal direction. Dorsal root ganglia may be left if a dorso-ventral dissection is to be performed; otherwise, remove them carefully.

7. Remove the dorsal half of **rat** spinal cord: lay the cord flat on a silicone support with its ventral face up, and cut along the middle of each side using a scalpel (*Figure 2D1*).

8. To remove the floor-plate from **chicken** spinal cord, hold one side of the cord with forceps and use microscissors to cut along the boundary between the floor-plate and the opposite side of the cord (*Figure 2D2*). Discard the side to which the floor-plate remains attached (it should be visible as a translucent fringe).

Protocol 2. Preparation of suspensions of dissociated spinal cord cells

1. Cut each cord into about 15 pieces using a scalpel.

2. Transfer the fragments to 10 ml plastic tubes in 1 ml of fresh CMF-PBS (the equivalent of two spinal cords per tube).

3. Add 20 µl of trypsin (2.5% w/v; final concentration 0.05%). Incubate for 15 min at 37 °C, agitating frequently.

4. Remove as much of the supernatant as possible using a 1 ml blue Gilson (or equivalent) tip, then add the following at room temperature:
   - culture medium (see *Table 3*)   0.8 ml
   - BSA (4% w/v; *Table 1*)   0.1 ml
   - DNase (1 mg/ml in L-15 medium; *Table 1*)   0.1 ml

5. Agitate vigorously by hand (3 min) until the DNase has digested the DNA that causes the tissue fragments to aggregate and until cells are spontaneously released into the medium (visible turbidity). Allow the remaining fragments to settle. Collect and pool the supernatants and then to each tube containing tissue fragments add:
   - culture medium   0.9 ml
   - BSA (4% w/v)   0.1 ml
   - DNase (1 mg/ml in L-15 medium)   20 µl

6. Immediately dilute the pooled supernatants twofold with L-15 medium and layer them gently on to a 1 ml cushion of BSA (4% w/v) in a 10 ml plastic centrifuge tube. Centrifuge for 10 min at 300 *g* at room temperature. Remove the supernatant containing trypsin and debris by aspiration from the surface. Resuspend the pellet in 1 ml culture medium by gentle passage through a Gilson blue tip; if DNA causes further aggregation, add 20 µl DNase solution.

7. During centrifugation of the BSA cushion, triturate the remaining tissue fragments by four gentle passages through a blue Gilson tip. Do not create bubbles or hold the tip close to the bottom of the tube. Allow the fragments to settle and pool the supernatants.

8. To each tube containing fragments, add medium and supplements as in step 5. Triturate eight times through a Gilson blue tip. Allow fragments to settle and pool supernatants. Little tissue should remain but, if necessary, repeat this step one more time. Discard any remaining tissue.

9. Pool all supernatants except that from step 6 and observe in a haemocytometer using a phase-contrast microscope. If there is much debris, pass the supernatants through a BSA cushion as described in step 6.

10. Pool all supernatants and observe under phase-contrast. Cells should be completely dissociated and ideally many will have neurites. The majority should be phase-bright, though the large motoneurons sometimes look quite grey as they flatten out in the haemocytometer (*Figure 3A*). Expect 1–2 x 10^6 cells/spinal cord.

Note: With E5 chicken spinal cords, steps 7–9 are often sufficient.

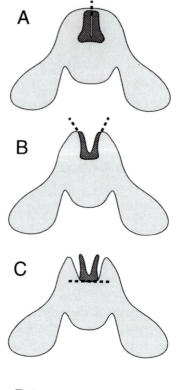

A

B

C

D1

D2

Figure 2. Dissection of embryonic spinal cord (see *Protocol 1*).

Protocol 3.   Metrizamide density gradient centrifugation
               (*Figure 1*)

1. Volumetrically prepare 6.5% (w/v) (for rat) and 6.8% (for chicken) solutions of metrizamide (Serva) in L-15 medium.

2. Put 2 ml of the appropriate metrizamide cushion into transparent polystyrene centrifuge tubes (one tube per four to five spinal cord equivalents). Layer the cell suspension dropwise on to the cushion,

holding the tube nearly horizontal. The interface should be sharp.

3. Centrifuge for 15 min at approx. 500 *g* (1600–2000 r.p.m.) in a bench-top centrifuge at room temperature. Vibration may be reduced by switching off the brake. There should be a pellet at the bottom of the tube (small cells) and a turbid band at the medium–metrizamide inter-face.

4. Remove the clear supernatant using a Gilson blue tip and collect the band in approx. 1 ml of medium, including some metrizamide at the interface. Dilute threefold with L-15 medium to lower the density, and collect the cells by centrifugation through a BSA cushion (*Protocol 2,* step 6).

5. Resuspend cells in 1 ml culture medium and observe under phase-contrast. The size distribution should be much narrower than before, with a predominance of large, round, phase-bright cells, and little debris (*Figure 3B*). Expect 50–70 000 cells per spinal cord, though this figure may be lower for E15 rat embryos.

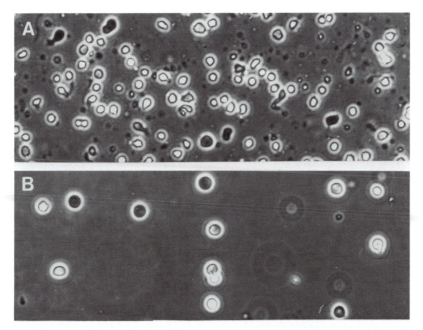

Figure 3. Typical aspect of cells in the haemocytometer. (A) Dissociated E5 chicken spinal cord; (B) motoneurons from same preparation after metrizamide and BSA cushions. Note relative enrichment for large cells. Scale bar as in *Figure 4A.*

Protocol 4. Immunopanning to purify motoneurons (*Figure 1*)

1. Incubate a 90 mm polystyrene bacteriological Petri dish (Greiner) overnight at 4 °C with the following (prepare one dish per four spinal cord equivalents). Ensure that the whole dish is covered:

   - 0.05 M Tris–HCl, pH 9.5   12 ml
   - affinity purified goat anti-mouse Ig antibody   10 µg

2. Rinse three times with 4 ml of CMF-PBS. Add 10 ml of the appropriate hybridoma supernatant at the indicated dilution in CMF-PBS:

   - (for chicken) SC1 monoclonal antibody   dilution 1 : 10
   - (for rat) IgG-192 monoclonal antibody   dilution 1 : 2

3. Incubate for 2 h at room temperature or (preferably) two days at 4 °C. Rinse three times with 4 ml of CMF-PBS. Do not allow to dry between washes. Add 10 ml of L-15 medium.

4. Add the cell suspension in culture medium and swirl the panning dish to distribute the cells evenly. Allow to stand for 40 min at room temperature. Observe in phase-contrast. When the dish is lightly tapped, unbound cells are seen to move. If a significant number of cells are bound, proceed with the next step. If not, wait another 20 min.

5. Swirl the dish and pour off the medium into a beaker. Wash three times gently with 4 ml L-15 medium, pouring the medium off and replacing immediately each time. Do not allow the dishes to stand without medium. Observe the dish: if cells are still strongly bound, do five more vigorous washes. If cells show signs of detachment, the washes may be stopped at this point.

6. Pour off the last wash from the dish and add 3 ml of undiluted hybridoma supernatant (SC1 for chicken, IgG-192 for rat) or 10 µg purified antibody dissolved in 3 ml L-15 containing 10% FCS. Holding the dish in one hand, tap it vigorously against the other palm so as to dislodge cells, continuing if necessary for 10 min. Do not allow dishes to stand at this stage, otherwise the centre will dry. When a majority of cells are detached, collect the medium using a Gilson blue tip. Replace with 3 ml of L-15 medium and apply a gentle stream of medium from a Gilson blue tip to all parts of the dish. Pool this medium with the first eluate and discard the panning dish.

7. Collect the purified motoneurons by centrifugation through a BSA cushion (*Protocol 2*, step 6). After a combination of metrizamide and immunopanning steps, expect 50 000 motoneurons per chicken spinal cord and 20 000 motoneurons per rat spinal cord.

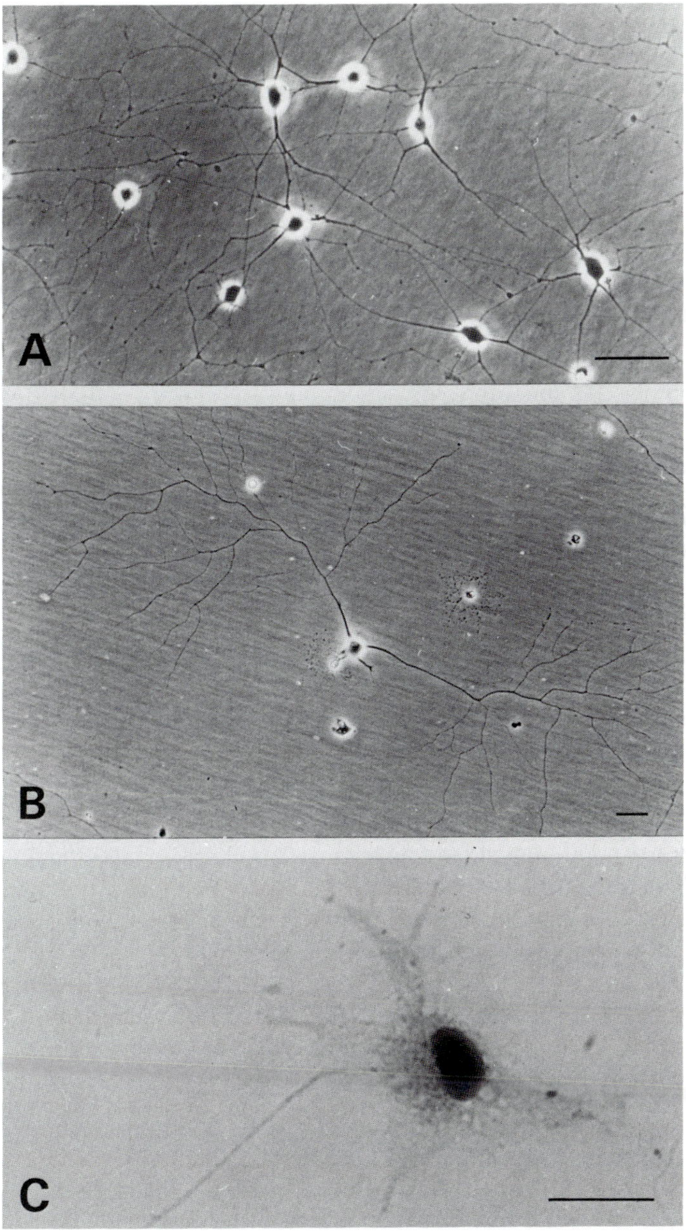

Figure 4. Motoneurons cultured for two days on laminin in the presence of growth pro-moting supplements. (A) E6 chicken motoneurons purified by metrizamide panning, grown at medium density in muscle extract. Scale bar, 50 μm. (B) An E14 rat moto-neuron grown at low density in 10 ng/ml LIF. Scale bar, 50 μm. (C) Nuclear labelling of an E15 rat motoneuron using a monoclonal antibody to Islet-1. Scale bar, 20 μm.

Protocol 5. **Culture of motoneurons**

1. Purified motoneurons from any of the previous protocols may be used immediately or stored for up to 48 h at 4 °C in the refrigerator in culture medium without bicarbonate (*Table 3*).

2. Coat tissue culture plastic with polyornithine-laminin (stock solutions in *Table 1*). Incubate dishes with polyornithine (diluted 1 : 1000 in water) at 20 °C for 30 min to overnight. Remove solution and allow to dry in hood. Add enough laminin (diluted 1 : 500 in L-15–bicarbonate) to well cover the surface of the dish. Incubate for 2 h to overnight at 37 °C in the CO_2 incubator.

3. Remove laminin and replace immediately with complete culture medium. Suitable growth promoting supplements depend on the species of motoneuron and on the experimental design. For chick, use muscle extract (see *Table 1* and ref. 7) diluted 1 : 300, which can be further supplemented with 10 ng/ml FGF-2 (basic fibroblast growth factor). For rat, use 100 pg/ml neurotrophin (BDNF, NT-3, or NT-4/5) and/or 10 ng/ml ciliary neurotrophic factor (CNTF) or leukaemia inhibitory factor (LIF).

4. Add motoneurons at a density appropriate for the experiment. Acute effects on cell survival are usually assayed at low density, whereas biochemical assays and long-term survival require higher density (refer to appropriate publications). Agitate dishes gently to ensure even distribution and put into incubator at 37 °C, saturating humidity, and 5% CO_2.

5. Neurite outgrowth should be extensive on laminin after the first night in culture (*Figure 4*). The purity of the culture may be confirmed using appropriate specific antibodies: SC1 or Islet-1 for chick; Ig-192 or Islet-1 for rat (*Figure 4*).

Acknowledgements

We thank our colleagues Sylvie Bouhanna, Annie Gouin, Bruno Hivert, and Clément Mettling for many useful hints and comments. This work was made possible by the generous gifts of antibody from: H. Tanaka (SC1), E. Johnson and P. Brachet (Ig-192), and S. Horton and T. Jessell (Islet-1). We were supported by the CNRS, the INSERM, the Association Française contre les Myopathies (AFM), and the Institut pour la Recherche sur la Moelle Epinière (IRME).

References

1. Camu, W., Bloch-Gallego, E., and Henderson, C. E. (1993). *Neuroprotocols*, **2,** 191.
2. Schnaar, R. L. and Schaffner, A. E. (1981). *J. Neurosci.*, **1,** 204.
3. Dohrmann, U., Edgar, D., and Thoenen, H. (1987). *Dev. Biol.*, **124,** 145.
4. Arakawa, Y., Sendtner, M., and Thoenen, H. (1990). *J. Neurosci.*, **10,** 3507.
5. Henderson, C. E., Camu, W., Mettling, C., Gouin, A., Poulsen, K., Karihaloo, M., *et al.* (1993). *Nature*, **363,** 266.
6. Bloch-Gallego, E., Huchet, M., El M'hamdi, H., Xie, F.-K., Tanaka, H., and Henderson, C. E. (1991). *Development*, **111,** 221.
7. Camu, W. and Henderson, C. E. (1992). *J. Neurosci. Meth.*, **44,** 59.
8. Tanaka, H. and Obata, K. (1984). *Dev. Biol.*, **106,** 26.
9. Yan, Q. and Johnson, E. J. (1988). *J. Neurosci.*, **8,** 3481.

II. CNS glia and non-neural cells

7

Astrocytes

DEREK R. MARRIOTT, WARREN D. HIRST, and M. CECILIA
LJUNGBERG

1. Introduction

The close anatomical association between astrocytes and neurons has long
been suggestive of some functional interplay between these cells. However,
the structural complexity of the CNS has often precluded definitive studies of
astrocytes *in vivo*. As a consequence the elucidation of their functional properties has relied, almost entirely, on tissue culture techniques. Cultured astrocytes are easily accessible to experimental manipulation and can now be
routinely prepared with greater than 95% homogeneity.

Primary astroglial cultures contain several morphologically and antigenically distinct forms of glial fibrillary acidic protein (GFAP)-positive astrocytes. The majority (type-1) are large, epithelioid cells which are labelled by
a monoclonal antibody against Ran-2, but are not labelled by the monoclonal
antibodies A2B5 and LB1 (against ganglioside antigens), or antibodies
against growth associated protein-43 (GAP-43). In contrast, most type-2
astrocytes have a stellate, process-bearing morphology, and in culture bind
A2B5, LB1, and antibodies against GAP-43, but not antibodies against Ran-2
(see refs 1–3). In addition, type-2 astrocytes and oligodendrocytes develop
from a bipotential O-2A progenitor cell, whereas type-1 astrocytes derive
from a different precurser cell (4). Studies have also shown that type-1 and
type-2 astrocytes also differ in a number of biochemical properties (5). Even
more studies have shown biochemical and functional differences between
type-1 astrocytes cultured from anatomically distinct regions of the CNS (6).

Virtually all of present techniques for the preparation of cultured astrocytes are based on the dissociation of neonatal tissue. Immature tissue is
more easily dissociated and yields more viable cells. Although not widely
used, procedures for isolating 'reactive' astrocytes from lesioned brain (7,8)
and astrocytes from dissociated adult tissue (9) have also been reported.
Traditionally, most methods have also used the general growth promoting
properties of serum to provide a mixture of hormones, growth factors, and
other nutritive substances. However, the constituents of serum are largely
undefined. Moreover, one batch can vary from another and serum con-

stituents can mask or alter the action of other compounds being examined (10). Although serum-free (defined) formulations for culturing neural tissue have been established for over a decade (11), only recently have studies using defined media begun to increase in the literature.

Here, we will describe methods to obtain and culture type-1 astrocytes from various regions of the immature rat CNS. In order to reflect recent trends, we have also incorporated a protocol for culturing astrocytes in defined growth medium and described a procedure for obtaining cells from the non-lesioned adult CNS. Finally, two methods are described for obtaining O-2A progenitor cells for differentiation into type-2 astrocytes. O-2A progenitor cells can be removed mechanically from the underlying astroglial monolayer and seeded directly into secondary culture (12). However, we have found that long-term cultures can contain variable proportions of microglia and type-1 astrocytes that have detached from the monolayer. Though initially not numerous, these cells rapidly divide and can, in long-term cultures, constitute more than 30% of the total cells present (13). Alternatively, the O-2A progenitor cells can be immunoselected by 'panning' from the cell suspension (see also Chapter 8 by Collarini). Whilst this reduces the yield, we have found that type-2 astrocyte cultures derived from immunoselected O-2A progenitor cells can approach 100% purity.

2. Mixed primary glial cultures

Astroglial cells cultured in serum-containing media will rapidly develop into a monolayer consisting predominantly of type-1 astrocytes. However, other glial and non-glial cells may also be present. We have found that fibroblasts can be particularly abundant in spinal cord cultures where the meninges are difficult to remove. This is circumvented by substituting D-valine for the L-isomer present in the normal culture media. D-Valine inhibits fibroblast growth as these cells lack the enzyme D-amino oxidase and are thus unable to utilize D-valine for growth (14).

Protocol 1. Mixed primary glial cell cultures from neonatal rat brain

Equipment and reagents

- Poly-L-lysine ($M_r > 300\,000$) (Sigma): prepare a 0.5 mg/ml stock solution in water, freeze in aliquots, and store at –20°C
- Earle's balanced salt solution (EBS) (Sigma): store at 4°C
- Deoxyribonuclease I (DNase I) (Sigma): store at –20°C
- Trypsin (type III, bovine fraction) (Sigma): store at –20°C
- Bovine serum albumin (BSA) fraction V (Sigma): store at 4°C
- Dulbecco's modified Eagles medium (DMEM) without L-valine and with L-glutamine, 187 mg/litre D-valine (Imperial Labs, No. 7–420–35), supplemented with 3.7 g/litre sodium bicarbonate—adjust to pH 7.6, filter sterilize, and store at 4°C

• D-Val DMEM: supplement DMEM with 0.33 mg/ml L-glutamine, 2.5% of antibiotic/antimycotic solution, and 10% (v/v) dialysed FCS. To remove serum L-valine from the FCS it is dialysed. Prepare dialysis tubing (dialysis membrane 9–36/32"; Medicell, 239 Liverpool Rd, London, UK), by boiling in four changes of 2% (w/v) sodium carbonate, 0.5% (w/v) EDTA. Rinse the tubing in water and dialyse the serum 1:50 (v/v) for three days, against three changes of 0.9% sodium chloride (w/v). Filter sterilize, aliquot, and store at –20 °C.

• D/L-Val DMEM: supplement the DMEM with 0.1 mg/ml L-valine, 0.33 mg/ml L-glutamine, 2.5% of antibiotic/antimycotic solution (v/v), and 10% (v/v) heat inactivated fetal calf serum (FCS), all from Sigma

Method

1. Make a solution of 5 µg/ml poly-L-lysine in water from the frozen stock. Filter sterilize the solution, cover the surface of the culture vessel, and incubate at 37 °C for 30–60 min. Aspirate the solution until the surfaces are completely dry and store in the hood until required. Poly-L-lysine is unstable in free solution but coated plastics etc. may be prepared in advance and stored in the hood.

2. Prepare a fresh solution of 4 mg of DNase and 0.3 g of BSA in 100 ml of EBS. Divide it into 2 x 50ml: to 1 x 50 ml add 12.5 mg of trypsin. Filter sterilize and heat to 37 °C.

3. We have found that P2 neonatal rat pups yield large numbers of viable cells with minimal cellular debris. Note however, that if cerebellum is to be cross-compared with other regions, cerebella should be obtained from P6 animals to maintain glial developmental equivalence. Sterilize all dissecting instruments in 70% ethanol and/or flame immediately prior to use. Kill the pups and remove and spray the head with 70% ethanol. Using fine dissecting scissors make two incisions from the vertebral canal across the ears and eyes, then lift and peel the skin and skull forward to reveal the cerebellum, cerebral cortices, and olfactory bulbs (*Figure 1A*).

4. (a) Cerebral cortices: using the curved forceps lift each hemisphere and cut the cortices between the midbrain and overlying cortex (*Figure 1B*).

   (b) Olfactory bulbs: sever the bulbs from the frontal cortex and remove with forceps.

   (c) Cerebellum: make two incisions, one vertical between the cerebellum and the brain, the other saggital (i.e. at a right angle to the first) between the cerebellum and the brain-stem.

   (d) Spinal cord: soak the body in 70% ethanol and make a small incision through the vertebral column at the base of the tail. Using fine scissors cut along the vertebral canal to the brown adipose tissue at the base of the neck. Using thumb and forefinger apply

Protocol 1. *Continued*

> pressure to both sides of the body to 'splay' open the vertebral column (*Figure 1C*). Insert the curved forceps near the base of the tail and gradually lift out the spinal cord. Grip the anterior end of the cord with forceps and sharply 'tug' it free from the neck (*Figure 1E*).

5. Into 1 x 50 ml tube per three cortices or an equivalent volume of tissue, place 15 ml of EBS/DNase/trypsin. Place the tissue into a 100 mm Petri dish containing about 0.5 ml of EBS/DNase/trypsin. Using a scalpel blade, finely chop the tissue twice, the second at right angles to the first, and add about 5 ml of the trypsin solution. Pipette the mixture into the 15 ml of EBS/DNase/trypsin and incubate at 37 °C, with gentle agitation for 15 min.

6. Add an equal volume of D/L-val DMEM to terminate trypsinization and spin at 250 *g*. Discard the supernatant and triturate the pellet about 20 times in 5 ml of EBS/DNase. Add a further 10 ml of EBS/DNase and allow the tissue to settle for about 10 min. Remove 10 ml of the supernatant into a 50 ml tube, taking care not to include any tissue from the bottom of the tube, and maintain at 37 °C. Add 2 ml of EBS/DNase to the tissue, triturate, and add another 10 ml of EBS/DNase. After 10 min remove the supernatant and add it to the first. Repeat this one more time then and spin at 250 *g* for 5 min.

7. Aspirate the supernatant and add 10 ml of D/L-val DMEM to the pellet. Using a 10 ml pipette gently disperse the pellet and then resuspend the tissue completely by triturating with a plugged glass Pasteur pipette. Make the volume up to 30 ml with D/L-val DMEM and count the cells. One pair of cortices or equivalent volume of tissue should be sufficient to plate a 175 cm^2 flask at a cell density of 2 x 10^5 cells/cm^2.

8. Incubate the cells in a 5% CO_2 incubator at 37 °C and change the culture medium after three days. After four or five days replace the D/L-val DMEM with D-val DMEM and change at three day intervals thereafter to retard the growth of fibroblasts and meningeal cells. The cultures should become confluent after approx. ten days.

Due to the relatively small number of cells in neonatal rat optic nerves, it is not feasible to bulk culture this region in large tissue culture vessels. Rather, this tissue should be cultured in small capacity multiwell plates or Lab-Tek chamber slides.

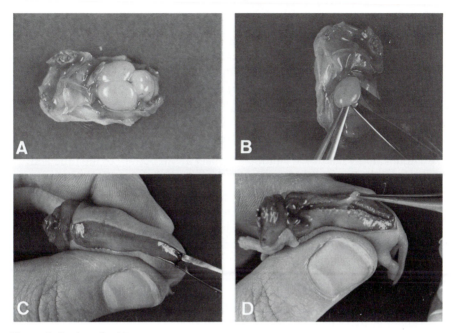

Figure 1. As described in text.

Protocol 2. Mixed primary glial cultures from neonatal rat optic nerves

Equipment and reagents
- EBS/DNase/trypsin, D/L-val DMEM, D-val DMEM, small dissecting scissors, fine forceps as in *Protocol 1*
- Dissecting microscope with fibre-optic illumination
- Multiwell plates (24-well) either with or without glass coverslips and/or Lab-Tek chamber slides (Nunc)

Method

1. Kill the rat pups and remove the eyes behind the eyeball with the fine scissors. Expose the cortex and olfactory bulbs as described in *Protocol 1*.

2. Remove the olfactory bulbs and place the head into a 10 cm Petri dish. Using a dissecting microscope, insert a microspatula at the front of the brain and lift the brain upward. The translucent optic nerves should be visible on the floor of the skull.

3. Still holding up the anterior part of the brain, insert a pair of forceps and grasp the nerves at the optic chiasm. Cut or 'pinch' the nerves free and transfer them to a Petri dish containing about 0.5 ml of EBS/DNase/trypsin.

Protocol 2. *Continued*

4. Dissect away any remaining optic chiasm and align the nerves in the same direction and, using a scalpel blade, finely chop the nerves at right angles to their long axis. Pipette the mixture into a 50 ml plastic tube containing 10 ml of EBS/DNase/trypsin and incubate at 37 °C for 15 min.

5. Let the tissue collect at the bottom of the tube and discard the supernatant. Wash the tissue twice in D/L-val DMEM and triturate about 20 times with a plugged Pasteur pipette.

6. Again, allow the tissue clumps to collect at the bottom of the tube and remove the supernatant to a centrifuge tube. Spin at 250 *g* for 5 min and resuspend the pellet in about 2.5 ml of D/L-val DMEM.

7. To plate the cells, seed 100 µl of the cell suspension into the middle of the glass coverslip (50 µl into a chamber slide) and transfer it to the incubator. After about 30 min flood the well with 0.5 ml of medium and culture as described in *Protocol 1*. The tissue from 30 optic nerves should yield sufficient cells to seed one 24-well multiplate or approx. six Lab-Tek chamber slides. After five to seven days the culture medium may be switched to D-val DMEM. The cultures should be confluent in 10–14 days.

As an alternative to serum-containing medium primary astroglial cultures can be maintained in a defined medium. We have evaluated a commercially available supplement (G-5 formulation) as a substitute for FCS. G-5 formulation contains insulin (5 mg/ml), transferrin (5.0 mg/ml), selenite (0.52 µg/ml), biotin (0.1 mg/ml), hydrocortisone (0.36 µg/ml), FGF (0.5 µg/ml), and EGF (0.1 µg/ml).

Protocol 3. Mixed primary astroglial cultures in serum-free media

Equipment and reagents
- Defined media: Ham's nutrient mixture F-12 (Imperial Labs), combined 1 : 1 with DMEM supplemented with 2.5% (v/v) antibiotic/antimycotic solution (Sigma) and 1% of 100 x G-5 formulation (Gibco): filter sterilize and store at 4 °C

Method

1. Prepare mixed primary astroglial cultures as described in *Protocol 1*.

2. If the cultures are to be seeded in defined medium the cell density should be about 4×10^5 cells/ml. Alternatively cells may be seeded at a density of 2×10^5 cells/ml in D/L-val DMEM for three days and then transferred to defined medium.

3. Defined medium should be changed after two days and at two day intervals thereafter.

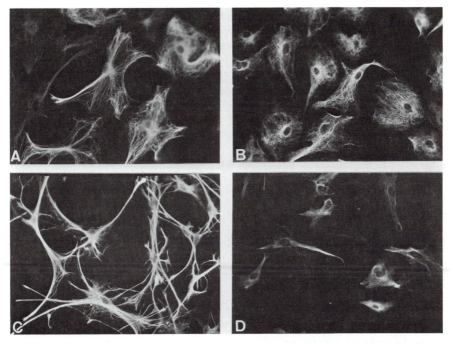

Figure 2. Immunofluorescent labelling of astrocyte enriched cultures with antibodies to GFAP. (A–C) Type-1 astrocytes derived from the cortices of P2 rat pups. The astrocytes were grown initially in D/L-valine DMEM containing 10% FCS and after four days changed to: (A) D-valine DMEM containing 10% dialysed FCS, (B) Ham's F-12 : DMEM (1 : 1) and maintained in the absence of serum, (C) Ham's F-12 : DMEM (1 : 1) supplemented with G-5 formulation. (D) Astrocytes derived from adult rat cortex.

After seven to ten days in either serum-containing or defined medium the cultures will have formed a monolayer consisting of more than 95% GFAP-positive type-1 astrocytes (*Figure 2A* and *B*). However, after approximately 24 hours the majority of cells cultured in defined media will adopt a stellate morphology (*Figure 2C*). Addition of dibutyryl cAMP to astroglial cultures is known to cause morphological conversion from flat to process-bearing cells (15). It is therefore likely that this stellate morphology reflects the presence of agents in G-5 which stimulate cAMP. It should be noted that whilst these cells remain antigenically identical to type-1 astrocytes, their functional equivalence with type-1 astrocytes cultured in serum-containing media is unknown.

3. Mixed primary astroglial cultures from *adult* tissue

We have used a modification of the method used for neonatal tissue to obtain astrocytes from the adult rat CNS. However, in our experience, the yield, purity, and identity of the cells thus obtained has proved problematic. Here, we describe a method for obtaining cells from dissociated adult midbrain, a proportion of which are GFAP-expressing astrocytes.

Protocol 4. Preparation of mixed primary astroglial cultures from adult tissue

Equipment and reagents

- Poly-L-lysine, EBS, DNase I, BSA, DMEM, D/L-val DMEM supplemented as in *Protocol 1*, fine scissors and forceps, and a dissecting microscope as described in *Protocols 1* and *2*
- Metal screen: 50 mesh (297 µm equivalent) and 200 mesh (74 µm equivalent) (Sigma)
- Cytosine 1-β-D-arabinofuranoside (AraC) (Sigma): make a stock solution of 10 mM AraC in DMEM, filter sterilize, aliquot, and store at −20°C
- 21G, 23G, and 25G needles
- EBS supplemented with 0.3% BSA as in *Protocol 1*
- Disposable cell scraper (Greiner)

Method

1. Coat tissue culture flasks in poly-L-lysine, prepare EBS solution with DNase and BSA as in *Protocol 1*.

2. Kill adult male Fisher rats weighing between 200 g and 250 g. Dissect the cortex and remove the meninges and blood vessels using a dissecting microscope.

3. Place the tissue into a 100 mm Petri dish (one cortex/dish) containing 0.5 ml of the EBS/DNase solution. With a scalpel blade, finely chop the tissue twice, the second at right angles to the first, then add about 10 ml of the EBS/DNase solution.

4. Transfer the mixture into a 50 ml tube and triturate the tissue about five times with a 5 ml pipette followed by five passages through a 21G needle. Filter the tissue through a 50 mesh screen and rinse with about 5 ml of the EBS/DNase solution. Triturate again with a 23G, needle followed by a 25G, needle and filter through a 200 mesh screen.

5. Spin at 250 *g* and resuspend the cells in about 45 ml of D/L-val DMEM. Counting of the cell suspension to determine the plating density is difficult as the mixture contains a large number of non-viable cells, myelin, and debris. In our experience one cortex is sufficient to plate three 75 cm² flasks.

6. Incubate the cells in a 5% CO_2 incubator at 37°C. Change the culture medium after two days and at three day intervals thereafter. Replacing the D/L-val DMEM with D-val DMEM (*Protocol 1*) does not inhibit

fibroblast proliferation in adult cultures, therefore we use another approach to tackle the problem of fibroblast contamination.

7. When cells become confluent (approx. three weeks) shake the flasks at 150 r.p.m. for 3 h to remove microglia. Aspirate the medium and add 20 ml of EBS containing 0.3% BSA. Using a disposable cell scraper remove the adherent cells, spin at 250 *g*, and resuspend and plate the cells in D/L-val DMEM. After 12–18 h treat the cells with two 48 h pulses of 10 μM AraC in D/L-val DMEM with a 24 h interval in between. Treatment with AraC kills fibroblasts which divide more rapidly than astrocytes.

8. The cultures can be maintained in D/L-val DMEM, or when confluent (approx. two weeks), subcultured as required.

In our experience the proportion of GFAP-expressing astrocytes (*Figure 2D*) can vary. It is possible that these cells are not astrocytic, or are astrocytes which have down-regulated GFAP.

4. Preparation of type-2 astrocytes

Mixed primary glial cultures can be optimized to promote the formation of O-2A progenitor cells. After about ten days these cultures will contain round, phase-bright microglia scattered diffusely on top of the monolayer and clonal groups of small, phase-dark, bipolar O-2A progenitor cells. Both cell types are removed from the astrocyte monolayer by mechanical shaking. The majority of the microglia are eliminated from the cell suspension by differential adhesion to untreated tissue culture plastic and oligodendrocytes are killed by complement-mediated cytolysis. The resulting suspension enriched in O-2A progenitors can then be seeded directly or further purified by immunoselection. The residual type-1 astrocyte monolayer may be further cultured in D-val DMEM, defined medium, and/or used as a source of type-1 astrocyte conditioned medium (15).

Protocol 5.   Enriched O-2A progenitor cells from mixed glial cultures

Equipment and reagents

- Incubator/shaker (PLS, East Grinstead, Sussex, UK), or a heated rotary shaker 2.5 cm throw, rated up to 250 r.p.m.
- D/L-Val DMEM as in *Protocol 1*, but containing 20% FCS
- 70 μm and 25 μm nylon mesh (Pharmacia): sterilized in 70% ethanol and air dried in the hood
- Anti-galactocebroside (GalC) (B. Ranscht)

Protocol 5. *Continued*

Method

1. Prepare mixed glial cultures as described in *Protocol 1* with the following modifications:

    (a)   Use P0 neonatal rats.

    (b)   Seed the cells at a density of 5 x 10⁴ cells/ml in 175 cm² tissue culture flasks.

    (c)   Add fresh D/L-val DMEM after 24 h and at three day intervals thereafter (we have noted that D-val DMEM can reduce the yield of O-2A progenitor cells).

2. Coat plastics/coverslips for the O-2A progenitor cells with 10 µg/ml poly-L-lysine for 30–60 min at 37 °C. Aspirate the solution until the flasks are completely dry.

3. Remove loosely adherent cells by 'pre-shaking' the flasks at 150 r.p.m. for 1 h at 37 °C. During this time the majority of the microglia will detach from the monolayer.

4. Aspirate the supernatant and replace with 30 ml per flask of D/L-val DMEM containing 20% FCS. Equilibrate the cultures in the incubator for approx. 2 h.

5. Remove the O-2A progenitor cells by shaking the flasks at 250 r.p.m. for 18 h at 37 °C. Filter the supernatant through the 60 µm and 100 µm gauze and spin at 250 *g* for 5 min. Resuspend the pellet in about 5 ml of EBS/DNase containing 10% normal rabbit serum as a source of complement and 20 µl of anti-GalC. Incubate at 37 °C for 60 min, wash in D/L-val DMEM, and spin at 250 *g* for 5 min. Plate the cells at a density of 10⁵ cells/ml. Cells thus obtained consist of approx. 80–90% O-2A progenitor cells.

As an alternative to direct plating of the cell suspension, O-2A progenitor cells can be immunopanned. This procedure utilizes the mouse monoclonal antibody LB1, which binds to the ganglioside GD3 present on O-2A progenitor cells.

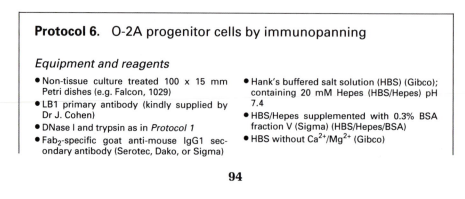

Protocol 6.   O-2A progenitor cells by immunopanning

Equipment and reagents

- Non-tissue culture treated 100 x 15 mm Petri dishes (e.g. Falcon, 1029)
- LB1 primary antibody (kindly supplied by Dr J. Cohen)
- DNase I and trypsin as in *Protocol 1*
- Fab₂-specific goat anti-mouse IgG1 secondary antibody (Serotec, Dako, or Sigma)
- Hank's buffered salt solution (HBS) (Gibco); containing 20 mM Hepes (HBS/Hepes) pH 7.4
- HBS/Hepes supplemented with 0.3% BSA fraction V (Sigma) (HBS/Hepes/BSA)
- HBS without Ca²⁺/Mg²⁺ (Gibco)

Method

1. Preparation of the panning dish: block non-specific binding sites with HBS/Hepes/BSA for 12–24 h. Aspirate the blocking solution and coat the dishes with 5–10 µg/ml of the secondary antibody diluted in HBS/Hepes for 12–24 h. (Note that the exact amount of antibody will depend on the batches of antibody and/or panning plates, therefore optimum titres should therefore be determined empirically by the experimenter.) A quantity of panning plates can be prepared and stored in blocking solution at 4 °C until required. Prepare one panning dish per four flasks of primary astrocytes.

2. Following shaking and collection of the cells by centrifugation (*Protocol 5*, step 5) resuspend the cells in 20 ml of HBS/Hepes containing 0.004% DNase I and 5 µg/ml (to be determined empirically) of LB1 primary antibody for 30 min, at 37 °C with gentle agitation. Spin for 5 min at 200 *g*, resuspend in approx. 7 ml of HBS/Hepes, and pipette the suspension into the panning dish.

3. Gently swirl the dish to obtain an even distribution and leave on a level non-vibrating surface for 10 min. Observe the cells under a dissecting microscope and gently agitate the solution. Adherent cells will consist of O-2A progenitors immobilized by the antibody and microglia sticking to the plastic.

4. To detach the microglia 'jarr' the side of the dish against a hard surface and aspirate the supernatant. To remove the antibody-immobilized cells, wash twice with HBS/Hepes and add approx. 7 ml of HBS without Ca^{2+}/Mg^{2+} containing 0.025% trypsin. Incubate for 5–10 min, occasionally 'jarring' the dish to remove the cells.

5. Transfer the cells into a centrifugation tube, wash the panning dishes twice with D/L-val DMEM and add to the tube. Spin at 250 *g* for 5 min and resuspend the pellet in approx. 2 ml of D/L-val DMEM. One flask should yield approx. 10^5 immunopanned cells. For type-2 astrocytes, the suspension should be seeded at a density of 2×10^5 cells/ml. Add fresh D/L-val DMEM after two to three days and at three day intervals thereafter.

After four days more than 98% of these cells are GFAP/GAP-43-positive type-2 astrocytes. These proportions should remain constant for at least 14 days.

Acknowledgements

This work was conducted in the laboratories of Drs Wilkin and Cohen. We would like to acknowledge support from the Wellcome Trust, SmithKline

Beecham Pharmaceuticals, and the University College Hospital Special Trustee's Fund.

References

1. Richardson, W. D., Raff, M., and Noble, M. (1990). *Semin. Neurosci.*, **2**, 445.
2. Curtis, R., Cohen, J., Fok-Seang, J., Hanley, M. R., Gregson, N. A., Reynolds, R., *et al.* (1988). *J. Neurocytol.*, **17**, 43.
3. Curtis, R., Hardy, R., Reynolds, R., Spruce, B. A., and Wilkin, G. P. (1991). *Eur. J. Neurosci.*, **3**, 876.
4. Raff, M. C., Miller, R., and Noble, M. (1983). *Nature*, **303**, 390.
5. Barres, B. A., Silverstein, B. E., Corey, D. P., and Chun, L. L. Y. (1988). *Neuron*, **1**, 791.
6. Wilkin, G. P., Marriott, D. R., and Cholewinski, A. J. (1990). *Trends Neurosci.*, **13**, 43.
7. Lindsay, R. M., Barber, P. C., Sherwood, M. R., Zimmer, J., and Raisman, G. (1982). *Brain Res.*, **243**, 329.
8. Trimmer, P. A. (1993). *Int. J. Dev. Neurosci.*, **11**, 125.
9. Schwartz, J. P. and Wilson, D. J. (1992). *Glia*, **5**, 75.
10. Romijn, H. J. (1988). *Biol. Cell*, **63**, 263.
11. Morrison, R. S. and De Vellis, J. (1981). *Proc. Natl. Acad. Sci. USA*, **78**, 7205.
12. McCarthy, K. and De Vellis, J. (1980). *J. Cell Biol.*, **85**, 890.
13. Marriott, D. R. and Wilkin, G. P. (1993). *J. Neurochem.*, **61**, 826.
14. Cholewinski, A. J., Reid, J. C., McDermott, A. M., and Wilkin, G. P. (1989). *Neurochem. Int.*, **15**, 365.
15. Gilad, G. M., Shanker, G., Dahl, D., and Gilad, V. H. (1990). *Brain Res.*, **508**, 215.

8

Oligodendrocyte lineage cells from neonatal rat brain

ELLEN J. COLLARINI

1. Introduction

Oligodendrocytes, the myelinating cells of the central nervous system, develop from precursor cells also known as O-2A progenitors because they can also be induced to develop into type-2 astrocytes *in vitro* (see Chp 7) (1). Although much is known about factors that influence the survival, proliferation, and differentiation of oligodendrocyte precursor cells (2–4), biochemical analyses of intracellular events that occur during the differentiation process have been hampered by the need for relatively large numbers of purified cells at various stages of development. In the last few years, however, several methods have been published that overcome this problem. Oligodendrocyte lineage cells have been obtained with varying degrees of purity from optic nerve (3), from neonatal rat brain (5,6), or from mixed glial cultures established from neonatal rat brain (7,8), using either density gradient separation (5) or variations on an immunoselective technique known as 'panning' (3,6–8), first described for isolating lymphocytes (9). In this technique, dishes are coated with antibodies against a particular cell/surface antigen, then the cell suspension is added to the dish to allow selective binding of cells that express that antigen.

The method described here uses mixed glial cultures as a starting point. When dissociated cells from cerebral hemispheres are cultured, they develop into a monolayer consisting mainly of astrocytes, with oligodendrocyte lineage cells on top of the monolayer (10). Cultures enriched in oligodendrocyte lineage cells can be obtained from mixed glial cultures by shaking them off the astrocyte monolayer (10) and re-plating the cells. Precursor cells can be further purified after shaking by a 'reverse panning' technique, in which the cells bind the antibody A2B5 in suspension, selectively preventing their attachment to Petri dishes (7). We have found that in our hands the yield and purity of oligodendrocyte precursor cells from mixed glial cultures can be improved by harvesting all the cells and then isolating the precursor cells by direct panning, using a modification of the technique used for isolating these cells from optic nerve (3). The cells can be maintained in a proliferative state with the complete suppression of differentiation by the addition of platelet-derived growth factor (PDGF) and basic fibroblast growth factor (bFGF) (11). By withdrawing growth factors the cells can be induced to differentiate more or less synchronously into oligodendrocytes, allowing the analysis of large populations of cells at approximately the same stage of differentiation. We have used this technique to obtain oligodendrocyte precursor cells in large enough quantities to analyse events occurring during oligodendrocyte differentiation at both the mRNA and protein levels (8).

2. Establishing mixed glial cultures

Mixed glial cultures are a convenient source of cells of the oligodendrocyte lineage. The cultures are established using modifications of the methods described by McCarthy and de Vellis (10) and Behar (7).

Protocol 1. Establishing mixed glial cultures from neonatal rat brain

Equipment and reagents

- Poly-D-lysine (M_r > 150 000) (Sigma): prepare 10 mg/ml 500 x stock in water, freeze in aliquots, and store at –20 °C
- 75 cm^2 tissue culture flasks or 10 cm tissue culture dishes
- Minimal essential medium buffered with 20 mM Hepes (MEM/Hepes) pH 7.4 (ICN)
- Deoxyribonuclease I (DNase I) (Sigma): prepare 0.4% (w/v) 100 x stock in PBS, filter sterilize, freeze in aliquots, and store at –20 °C

- Curved scissors, straight forceps, curved No. 7 jeweller's forceps, scalpel or razor blade
- 60 µm nylon mesh (Plastok Associates, Birkenhead, Merseyside, UK), sterilized with 70% EtOH and air dried in the hood
- Dulbecco's modified Eagle's medium (DMEM; ICN) supplemented with 4 mM glutamine, 100 U/ml penicillin, 100 µg/ml streptomycin, and 10% fetal calf serum (DMEM/10% FCS)

Method

1. Make up a solution of 20 µg/ml poly-D-lysine in sterile water from frozen stock. Add approx. 5 ml to each flask or dish. Leave to coat the dish for at least 30 min, aspirate, and then leave open in the tissue culture hood to dry completely.

2. Kill and decapitate new-born rat pups (one-day-old), place head on a board, and anchor down with pin or needle at the nose and through the skin at the back of the head. Spray with 70% ethanol and allow to dry. From this point on, work under sterile conditions. Using curved scissors, cut the skin, and then the skull, from between and in front of the eyes, out to the side towards the ears (*Figure 1A*). Lift up on the scissors while cutting the skull to avoid cutting into the brain. Pull back and pin down the flaps of skin and skull to expose the brain. Use

the curved forceps to cut and lift out the brain. Place brains into 60 mm Petri dishes (two brains/dish) with enough MEM/Hepes to cover them.

3. Using forceps under a dissecting microscope, remove any of the olfactory bulbs that may still remain attached (*Figure 1B*). Use forceps, razor blade, or scapel to bisect the brain along the midline into two hemispheres. Turn one hemisphere over (ventral side up) and slip one arm of the curved forceps between the cortex and overlying structures on either side; this gap is visible on the medial side (see *Figure 1C*). Press down slightly and squeeze the arms of the forceps together to clip away the overlying tissue. Most of the overlying tissue can be removed with this one operation; clean away any other overlying tissue, and use the forceps to remove the hippocampus (*Figure 1D*). The remaining shell of tissue consists of cerebral cortex and underlying white matter. Turn the shell over (convex side up). Using two curved forceps, hold the shell of tissue steady with the blunt curve of one closed pair of forceps (you need to use some downward pressure, but be careful not to crush the tissue), and take hold of the meninges with the tips of the other; there is usually a loose flap of meninges somewhere with which to start. Gently pull the sheet of meninges away from the cortex (*Figure 1D*). When the meninges have been completely removed, transfer the hemisphere of tissue to a clean dish containing MEM/Hepes. Continue until all hemispheres have been cleaned.

4. Aspirate the medium from the dish containing the hemispheres. Use the curved scissors to cut up the tissue into a fine 'mush', making sure no large fragments of tissue remain. Resuspend the minced tissue in a few millilitres of MEM/Hepes and transfer to a small vial with a Pasteur pipette, in a final volume of about 5–7 ml MEM/Hepes for ten brains. Add DNase I from a frozen 100 x stock to a final concentration of 0.004% (w/v). Pull the tissue suspension slowly through a syringe fitted with a 19G needle, then push the suspension back into the vial. Repeat this operation, changing to a 21G, a 23G, and finally a 25G needle. This operation needs to be done very slowly for best recovery. The small air bubble that rests under the plunger of the syringe serves as an indicator; push or pull with just enough pressure to avoid visibly distorting the bubble.

5. Filter the cell suspension through the sterile 60 μm nylon mesh into a 15 ml tube, using more MEM/Hepes to rinse out the vial and mesh. Top up the tube with MEM/Hepes, and spin at 200 *g* for 5–7 min. Aspirate the supernatant, resuspend the pellet in DMEM/10% FCS, fill the tube to the top with DMEM/10% FCS, and spin again.

6. Resuspend pellet in DMEM/10% FCS and split into the poly-D-lysine coated 75 cm² flasks or 10 cm dishes in a final volume of 10 ml of

Protocol 1. *Continued*

DMEM/10% FCS/flask or dish. The cell density should be about 1.5 × 10^7/flask, approx. one to one and one-half brains/flask or dish. Swirl the flasks/dishes to get even distribution, and incubate in a 5% CO_2 incubator at 37 °C. An hour or so later, give the flasks/dishes a swirl to redistribute the cells.

7. Two to three days later, wash the flasks/dishes to remove most of the debris (tap firmly to dislodge the debris from the surface), and replace with fresh DMEM/10% FCS. The medium should then be changed every two to three days.

After seven or eight days, the cultures will develop into a monolayer consisting mainly of astrocytes, with small, phase-dark, process-bearing cells on top of the monolayer that will visibly increase in number over the last few days in culture. The cells on top include oligodendrocyte lineage cells, and at this stage the cells are ready for harvesting.

3. Isolation of oligodendrocyte precursor cells from mixed glial cultures

Cultures enriched for oligodendrocytes and precursors can be obtained by shaking the flasks on a rotary shaker and then re-plating the detached cells (10), or by further purification by immunoselection (7). We have found that trypsinizing the cells and then panning, based on the method of Barres *et al.* (3), gives a higher yield and purity of cells.

Panning dishes are used to remove most of the major contaminating cells, astrocytes and meningeal cells, and the differentiated oligodendrocytes. Astrocytes and meningeal cells are removed using dishes coated with antibody to RAN-2 (12), and oligodendrocytes using dishes coated with antigalactocerebroside (GalC) (13). Macrophages are also removed during these two steps by virtue of binding via their Fc receptors to the antibody-coated dishes. Finally, oligodendrocyte precursor cells are positively selected on dishes coated with the monoclonal antibody A2B5 (14).

Protocol 2. Preparation of panning dishes

The day before harvesting the cells, set-up the panning dishes. First, goat anti-mouse IgG or IgM is bound to the plastic, then the cell-specific antibody is added.

Equipment and reagents

- Goat anti-mouse IgG or IgM (Sigma or Jackson Laboratories): prepare 1–2 mg/ml stocks, freeze in aliquots, and store at −20 °C

- Primary antibodies: RAN-2 (12) (American Type Culture Collection), GalC (13) (also, antibody available from Cedarlane Laboratories or Sigma—not tested by author), and A2B5 (14) (ATCC)

- 50 mM Tris buffer pH 9.0
- Falcon Petri dishes (NOT tissue culture plastic), either 100 mm or 150 mm
- MEM/20 mM Hepes with 0.2% bovine serum albumin (BSA), fraction V (Sigma)

Method

1. Set up panning dishes with the first antibody: for RAN-2 and GalC antibodies use goat anti-mouse IgG, and for A2B5 use goat anti-mouse IgM. Use these antibodies at 10 μg/ml. Dilute the antibodies in 50 mM Tris pH 9, add to dishes, swirl until dishes are completely covered with the solution, and store at 4°C for 4 h to overnight. 100 mm dishes require approx. 7 ml volume, 150 mm dishes require 14 ml. For ten flasks of mixed glial cell cultures, make up ten RAN-2 dishes, five GalC dishes, and five A2B5 dishes if using 100 mm dishes; make six RAN-2 dishes, three GalC dishes, and three A2B5 dishes if using 150 mm dishes.

2. The next day, wash the panning dishes three times with PBS, and then add the cell-specific antibody in MEM/Hepes with 0.2% BSA. Use monoclonal supernatants at a dilution between 1 : 5 and 1 : 10 or ascites at approx. 1 : 3000 (determined empirically). A2B5 must be at a concentration that will cause cell attachment, but will also allow cells to be removed from the panning dish by trypsin.

3. Leave for at least 1 h, and leave on until dishes are ready to be used.

Protocol 3. Panning oligodendrocyte precursor cells

Equipment and reagents

- Trypsin (Sigma): 100 x stock of 2.5% (w/v), frozen in aliquots
- Trypsin inhibitor (Sigma): prepare 100 x stock of 2.5% (w/v) soybean trypsin inhibitor and 0.4% DNase I (w/v) in Ca^{2+}/Mg^{2+}-free buffer, filter sterilize, and freeze in aliquots
- DMEM without Ca^{2+}/Mg^{2+} or balanced salt solution without Ca^{2+}/Mg^{2+}
- MEM supplemented with 20 mM Hepes (MEM/Hepes)
- DNase I (same as that used in *Protocol 1*)
- 20 μm nylon mesh (Plastok Assoc, Birkenhead, Merseyside, UK), sterilized with 70% EtOH and air dried in the hood
- Basic fibroblast growth factor (bFGF) (Peprotech, New Jersey, USA): 2 μg/ml stock in 1 mg/ml BSA; store aliquots at –70°C.

- Heat inactivated fetal calf serum (incubate at 55°C, 30 min)
- DMEM supplemented with BSA (0.1 mg/ml), insulin (5 μg/ml), human transferrin (0.1 mg/ml), putrescine (16 μg/ml), progesterone (60 ng/ml), sodium selenite (40 ng/ml), thyroxine (40 ng/ml), and tri-iodothyronine (30 ng/ml), a modification of Bottenstein and Sato (15) defined medium (referred to as B-S medium)—all supplements are Sigma cell culture reagents
- Platelet-derived growth factor, AA homodimer (PDGF-AA) (Peprotech, New Jersey, USA): 2 μg/ml stock in 10 mM acetic acid and 1 mg/ml BSA; store aliquots at –70°C
- Tissue culture dishes and/or coverslips coated with poly-D-lysine as described in *Protocol 1*

Method

1. Wash cells three times with Ca^{2+}/Mg^{2+}-free DMEM (DMEM–CM) or buffered salt solution without Ca^{2+}/Mg^{2+}. Add 2 ml DMEM–CM and

Protocol 3. *Continued*

20 µl trypsin stock. Incubate for about 5 min with occasional swirling, until most cells come off the flask when tapped. Antibody staining of cells and selective adhesion of cells to antibody-coated plates indicate that this brief trypsinization does not destroy the antigenic determinants used in this procedure.

2. While cells are in the incubator, make up the trypsin inhibitor from 100 x stock with DMEM–CM and add approx. 2 ml to 15 ml centrifuge tubes. For ten flasks of cells use four tubes.

3. Transfer cells to centrifuge tubes with trypsin inhibitor. Rinse each flask with a few millilitres of the inhibitor solution and add to tubes. Spin for 5 min at 150 *g*.

4. Aspirate supernatant and gently resuspend pellets with about 1 ml of the trypsin inhibitor using a blue Gilson tip. Top up the tubes with DMEM–CM and spin again for 5 min. Repeat this two more times. The repeated washing in Ca^{2+}/Mg^{2+}-free buffer helps to further dissociate the cells; the pellets should resuspend more easily with each wash.

5. Resuspend in 0.5 ml of trypsin inhibitor. Add 0.5 ml MEM/Hepes and gently triturate a few times. Top up the tubes with MEM/Hepes and spin for 5 min.

6. During the spins prepare MEM/Hepes with 0.5% heat inactivated FCS and 0.004% DNase I. The volume will depend on the size and number of plates you are using; for ten flasks use approx. 20 ml to split between five 100 mm RAN-2 dishes or 24 ml for three 150 mm RAN-2 dishes.

7. Resuspend the cells in the MEM/Hepes solution, combining all cells into one tube. Filter the cell suspension through the 20 µm nylon mesh into another tube.

8. Wash the first set of panning dishes (one-half the RAN-2 dishes) three times with PBS, and evenly distribute the cells to these dishes. The density will be approx. 3×10^7 cells/150 mm dish. Swirl well to get an even distribution, and leave undisturbed on a level, non-vibrating surface for 20–30 min.

9. Wash next set of dishes (the rest of the RAN-2 dishes). Swirl first set of dishes a few times to get the non-adherent cells into suspension, and transfer cells to the next set, taking care to recover all the medium from the first set (stand the dishes on their sides against the wall of the hood to allow medium to drain to bottom). Leave cells for 30 min.

10. Continue as above, transferring cells to the GalC then the A2B5 dishes. After 30 min on the A2B5 dishes (positive selection step), carefully wash the dishes with 6–8 ml MEM/Hepes until no floating

cells remain (at least ten times). Wash the dishes by holding them at a 45° angle, aiming the pipette towards the side of the dish, and slowly ejecting the liquid while moving the pipette tip back and forth along the side. The medium will run down the dish and should cover the surface. Collect the medium from the bottom of the dish. Finally, wash two to three times with DMEM–CM, add 3 ml (100 mm dishes) or 6 ml (150 mm dishes) DMEM–CM, and trypsin at 0.025%. Incubate about 10 min, or until tapping the dish loosens most of the cells. The rest of the cells can then be removed by washing the surface repeatedly with the trypsin solution. Transfer cells to 15 ml centrifuge tubes, wash the dishes with DMEM supplemented with 10% heat-inactivated FCS, and add to the tubes. Spin for 10 min at 200 *g*.

11. While the cells are spinning, add the B-S medium to the poly-D-lysine coated dishes that will receive the cells. Put in the incubator to adjust temperature and pH.

12. Combine cell pellets if necessary and wash cells once more in DMEM/10% FCS. Resuspend cells in DMEM/10% FCS and add to the dishes, along with any additional growth factors, in a volume that gives a final FCS concentration of 0.5%. The yield should be $1-2 \times 10^6$ from ten 75 cm² flasks. Plate the cells at a density of 5×10^5 on 6 cm dishes. The addition of bFGF and PDGF-AA (both at maximal mitogenic activity, usually 5–10 μg/ml), will allow these cells to proliferate and prevent differentiation (11). Supplement bFGF every day and PDGF-AA every other day (7).

After 48 h in growth factors, 98% or more of these cells are A2B5 positive (see *Figure 2*), with 2–3% of them also expressing GalC. When growth factors are removed, GalC expression increases over several days. If the cells are plated in the absence of growth factors, at least 95% express GalC within 48 h (see *Figure 2*). 1–3% of the cells in these cultures are positive for glial fibrillary acidic protein.

Acknowledgements

I am deeply indebted to Professor William Richardson, in whose laboratory this work was done, not only for comments on the manuscript, but also for his support, advice, and encouragement. I am also grateful for advice from Barbara Barres on panning and for the assistance of Caroline Marshall during the development of these procedures. This work was funded by a grant from the Medical Research Council.

A.   cut skin and skull along lines indicated:

B.   split brain into two halves and remove olfactory bulbs:

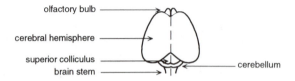

olfactory bulb

cerebral hemisphere

superior colliculus

brain stem

cerebellum

C.   remove brain stem, cerebellum, diencephalon and striatum
from cerebral hemisphere:

single hemisphere, ventral side up:

cortex

diencephalon
(hypothalamus, thalamus)
and striatum

brain stem (including colliculi)
and cerebellum

curved forceps

D.   remove hippocampus and meninges

ventral side up: ventral side down:

cortex

hippocampus

meninges

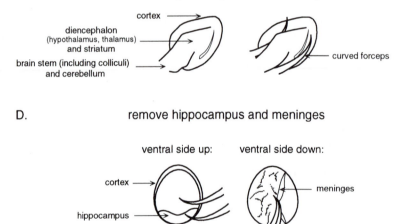

Figure 1. Dissection guide. (A) Cut the skin and then the skull along the lines indicated, and remove the brain. (B) Split the brain into two hemispheres and remove the olfactory bulbs. (C) With the ventral side up, separate the overlying tissue from the hemisphere. (D) Remove the hippocampus. Turn the hemisphere over (ventral side down) and gently peel off the meninges.

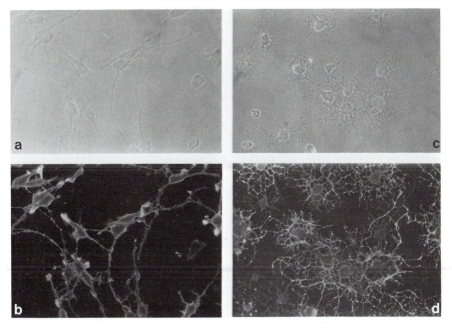

Figure 2. Cultures of purified oligodendrocyte lineage cells. Photographs of purified oligodendrocyte precursor cells grown for 48 h in medium containing PDGF-AA and bFGF (a and b) or without additional growth factors (c and d). The cells cultured with growth factors are shown (a) in phase-contrast and (b) stained with A2B5 followed by a fluorescent antibody. The cells cultured without growth factors are shown (c) in phase-contrast and (d) stained for GalC followed by a fluorescent antibody.

References

1. Raff, M. C., Miller, R. H., and Noble, M. (1983). *Nature*, **303**, 390.
2. Richardson, W. D., Raff, M., and Noble, M. (1990). *Semin. Neurosci.*, **2**, 445.
3. Barres, B. A., Hart, I. K., Coles, H. S. R., Burne, J. F., Voyvodic, J. T., Richardson, W. D., *et al.* (1992). *Cell*, **70**, 31.
4. Barres, B. A. and Raff, M. C. (1994). *Neuron.*, **12**, 935.
5. Lubetzki, C., Goujet-Zalc, C., Gansmüller, A., Monge, M., Brillat, A., and Zalc, B. (1991). *J. Neurochem.*, **56**, 671.
6. Gard, A. L. and Pfeiffer, S. E. (1989). *Development*, **106**, 119.
7. Behar, T., McMorris, F. A., Novotny, E. A., Barker, J. L., and Dubois-Dalcq, M. (1988). *J. Neurosci. Res.*, **21**, 168.
8. Collarini, E. J., Kuhn, R., Marshall, C. J., Monuki, E. S., Lemke, G., and Richardson, W. D. (1992). *Development*, **116**, 193.
9. Wysocki, L. J. and Sato, V. L. (1978). *Proc. Natl. Acad. Sci. USA*, **75**, 2844.
10. McCarthy, K. D. and de Vellis, J. (1980). *J. Cell Biol.*, **85**, 890.
11. Bögler, O., Wren, D., Barnett, S. C., Land, H., and Noble, M. (1990). *Proc. Natl. Acad. Sci. USA*, **87**, 6368.

12. Bartlett, P. F., Noble, M. D., Pruss, R. M., Raff, M. C., Rattray, S., and Williams, C. A. (1981). *Brain Res.*, **204,** 339.
13. Ranscht, B., Clapshaw, P. A., Price, J., Noble, M., and Seifert, W. (1982). *Proc. Natl. Acad. Sci. USA*, **79,** 2709.
14. Eisenbarth, G. S., Walsh, F. S., and Nirenburg, M. (1979). *Proc. Natl. Acad. Sci. USA*, **76,** 4913.
15. Bottenstein, J. E. and Sato, G. H. (1979). *Proc. Natl. Acad. Sci. USA*, **76,** 514.

Microglia: the tissue macrophage of the CNS

M. NICOLA WOODROOFE and M. LOUISE CUZNER

1. General introduction

Microglia are distinct from neurons and macroglia and are of probable meso-dermal origin. Monocytes/macrophages infiltrate the central nervous system (CNS) during development and in the adult animal take on the ramified morphology of resting microglia, no longer expressing the full complement of macrophage markers (1). Microglia are present in all brain areas but are not uniformly distributed, being enriched in grey matter (2). In the mouse brain the proportion varies from 5% in the cortex to 12% in the substantia nigra. The morphology of microglia *in vivo* varies according to their location and microenvironmental factors and ranges from compact amoeboid cells to ramified, branched cells, with considerable variation in the length and complexity of branching of the processes. Their plasticity is emphasized by their rapid morphological changes in response to mechanical or pathological insults.

Although the consensus at present is that microglia originate in the bone marrow the development of cell-specific markers which could distinguish microglia from other subpopulations of macrophages would significantly contribute to studies of their ontogeny. Such markers would also distinguish between resident macrophages which traffic between the CNS and the circulation. Microglia share many if not most of the characteristics and properties of other macrophage populations and *in vitro* studies have highlighted brain-specific features. Microglia can be isolated and maintained *in vitro* where their external environment can be manipulated and the resultant effect on microglial properties determined, thus furthering our understanding of the functional role of microglia in health and disease. In culture microglia can adopt three distinct morphologies: amoeboid, bipolar, and ramified, process-bearing cells, similar to those seen *in vivo*. The procedures for isolating microglia may themselves result in a certain degree of cell activation and this must be taken into account when *in vitro* phenotypic and functional studies are undertaken.

2. Isolation of microglia

2.1 Introduction

Mechanical and/or enzymatic dissociation of brain tissue yields a cell suspension of which microglia comprise a correspondingly small number. In order to obtain a pure population of microglia, 'contaminating' cells must be eliminated. Whilst culture conditions can be selected such that neuronal cell survival is prohibited, it has been necessary to devise methods for separation of microglia from macroglial cells. The differential ability of the cells to adhere under various culture conditions can be used to advantage in isolating microglia, as in a method described originally by McCarthy and de Vellis (3). More recently this laboratory has exploited the surface expression of Fc receptors on microglia to isolate the cells by density gradient centrifugation following rosetting with opsonized erythrocytes (4), while a third method uses density gradient centrifugation alone to separate microglia from mixed glia (5). All procedures involve monitoring of the isolated cells with macrophage-specific monoclonal antibodies or lectins as well as ensuring that cells expressing glial fibrillary acidic protein (GFAP) and galactocerebroside (GalC) (markers of astrocytes and oligodendrocytes respectively) are absent. A criticism levelled at microglial isolates concerns the proportion of contaminating monocytes, which is difficult to assess since as mentioned previously, identifying markers are common to both macrophages and microglia. This problem was addressed in our laboratory by counting the numbers of contaminating erythrocytes in the initial mixed glia population which permits a theoretical calculation of the number of contaminating monocytes (4). Perfusion of the animal before removing the brain will reduce the number of contaminating monocytes in the brain cell isolates.

Microglia have been isolated from a number of different species, at different ages of development including human adult (4,6) and fetal brain (7), rat brain at all developmental stages (4,8,9), and neonatal mouse brain (10,11). Consideration should be given to the age of the animal from which microglia are isolated since adherence properties of the glial cells at different developmental stages are distinct. For example, human fetal microglia are less adherent and adult microglia more adherent than astrocytes (6,7). Similarly, in this laboratory, adult human microglia have been found to be more adherent than oligodendrocytes (12). Thus care must be taken at each stage to check on the population of cells which detaches and those that remain adherent. Certain general procedures are followed for the cell isolation, all under conditions of sterility. The tissue, most usually the forebrain in animal species and corpus callosum from human white matter, is dissected and the meninges and visible blood vessels removed either with forceps or by rolling the brain on filter paper. The tissue can then be processed by the methods outlined below to separate the microglia.

2.2 Dissociation of CNS tissue

CNS tissue is dissociated mechanically with or without accompanying enzyme digestion, resulting in a mixed glia suspension from which the microglia are separated. Mechanical dissociation of the brain tissue is carried out by chopping or by trituration alone, as in the case of fetal rat brain and through sieves or nylon meshes for adult brain. Generally mechanical dissociation is followed by an enzyme digestion step to enhance disaggregation. Trypsin (0.25%) and DNase (50 µg/ml) are commonly used and in our laboratory collagenase is also included. The enzyme digestion is usually carried out at 37 °C for up to 1 h. DNase is necessary to disrupt the DNA, released as a result of the tissue dissociation, which would otherwise result in a gelatinous mixed glial cell suspension which is difficult to process further. The enzymes are neutralized by adding serum to the suspension and the cells are centrifuged and in some cases filtered through nylon mesh. After washing, the mixed glial cell suspension is ready for further manipulation to allow separation of the microglia.

2.3 Separation of microglia

Three techniques have been reported for the separation of microglia from mixed glial cell suspensions and are summarized in *Figure 1*. The most widely used of these methods is the shaking procedure.

2.3.1 Rosetting method (4)

Microglia are obtained by incubating the mixed glia with opsonized human erythrocytes (prepared by adding rabbit anti-human erythrocyte antibody to freshly isolated human red cells). The rosetted microglia (shown in *Figure 3a*) are then separated from other cells and any contaminating myelin, by density gradient centrifugation. The rosetted microglia form a pellet at the bottom of the tube while the interface contains myelin and other glial cells. The pellets are collected and subjected to hypotonic lysis to remove bound erythrocytes. After repeating the hypotonic lysis step, cells are counted and plated out.

Protocol 1.   Preparation of opsonized human erythrocytes

- 50 ml Falcon tubes
- Rabbit anti-human erythrocyte antibody (Dako)
- EBSS plus Ca/Mg plus pen–strep
- Human blood

This method can be used for both antibody coating or complement coating of erythrocytes

Method

1. Collect human peripheral venous blood by venepuncture into heparinized tubes.

2. Centrifuge the blood at 200 *g* for 10 min.

Protocol 1. *Continued*

3. Remove the plasma and resuspend the cells in EBSS plus Ca/Mg.

4. Pellet cells and carefully remove the buffy coat layer above the red cell pellet.

5. Wash the cells in EBSS.

6. Make a 2% (v/v) suspension of erythrocytes (RBCs) by adding 1 ml of packed RBCs to 49 ml EBSS.

7. Add antibody against human red cells at 1/600 dilution and incubate on a rotator for 30 min at room temperature. (A subagglutinating concentration of antibody is selected.)

8. Wash coated red cells (EA) twice and resuspend to the original volume to give a 2% EA suspension.

Protocol 2. Microglial cell isolation

Equipment and reagents

- McIlwain tissue chopper (The Mickle Laboratory Engineering Co., Mill Works, Gomshall, Surrey)
- Earle's balanced salt solution ± Ca/Mg (Gibco, Cat. No. 04104015 and 04104155)
- Dulbecco's modified Eagle medium (Gibco, Cat. No. 04101965)
- Penicillin–streptomycin (pen–strep, 100 × concentrate) (Gibco, Cat. No. 04305140)
- Fetal calf serum
- Trypsin (Sigma, type III)
- Collagenase (Sigma, type IV)
- DNase I (Sigma, type II)
- New-born calf serum
- Nylon mesh pore size 80 μm and 132 μm (J. Staniar and Co., UK)
- Percoll (Pharmacia)
- Sterile distilled water
- BME Hank's without L-glutamine 10 × concentrate (Gibco, Cat. No. 04201521)
- Sterile glass bottles (Duran type) and magnetic stir bars
- Tissue culture plastics—10 ml sterile pipettes, 50 ml Falcon tubes, Petri dishes (90 mm) (Gibco)
- 8-well chamber slides (Lab Tech, ICN Biologicals, UK)
- Culture medium: to 450 ml DMEM add 50 ml of heat inactivated fetal calf serum and 5 ml of stock pen–strep (C-DMEM); add 5 ml pen–strep to 500 ml EBSS solution
- Enzyme stock solutions (prepare stock enzyme solutions in EBSS plus Ca/Mg): trypsin (1.25% w/v), collagenase (1000 U/ml), and DNase I (100 μg/ml), pass through 0.22 μm filters to sterilize and store in 10 ml aliquots at –20 °C—these are 10 × final concentrations

The protocol is given for 10 g of brain tissue (ten rats) and all procedures are carried out under sterile conditions and at 4 °C using ice or refrigeration, unless indicated otherwise.

1. Chop brain tissue in two 90° planes in 0.4 mm slices on a McIlwain chopper and weigh 10 g of tissue into a sterile glass bottle.

2. For the enzymatic dissociation, add 10 ml of each stock enzyme solution (trypsin, DNase, and collagenase) together with 70 ml EBSS plus Ca/Mg at 37 °C, and incubate the mixture with stirring at 37 °C for 15 min.

3. Divide the mixture between six 50 ml Falcon tubes and add 10 ml

new-born calf serum to each tube, and top up with 15 ml EBSS minus Ca/Mg. Centrifuge at 140 g, for 10 min.

4. Transfer the pellets back to the bottles and repeat the enzyme digestion procedure (steps 2 and 3).

5. Resuspend the pellet in EBSS plus Ca/Mg and pass through 132 μm and 80 μm nylon mesh using the plunger of a syringe to push the mixture through (see *Figure 2*). Make up to 50 ml with EBSS plus Ca/Mg.

6. Count the brain cells and erythrocytes using a haemocytometer.

7. Percoll preparation. Adjust the Percoll density to 1.086 g/ml by adding 10 x HBS and sterile distilled water in the ratio 62 ml Percoll : 28 ml H_2O : 10 ml 10 x HBS.

8. Mix the mixed glial cell suspension, resuspended to 50 ml in EBSS plus Ca/Mg, with an equal volume of EA. Incubate the mixture at 37 °C for 30 min, centrifuge, and gently resuspend the pellet to the original volume in EBSS minus Ca/Mg.

9. Overlay 25 ml of glia/EA mixture on to 25 ml 1.086 g/ml Percoll (gradient) and centrifuge at 700 g for 20 min at room temperature, without the brake on.

10. Resuspend the pellets containing both rosetted cells and EA in 5 ml EBSS minus Ca/Mg and quickly add 39 ml of ice-cold sterile H_2O in a 50 ml tube. Gently shake the tube for 30 sec and then restore tonicity by adding 5 ml of 10 x BME Hank's. Pellet the cells and repeat this cold hypotonic lysis step to remove the RBCs.

11. Plate cells for culture at 2 x 10^5 cells/well in tissue culture chamber slides or in 96-well flat-bottomed plates (10^5 cells/150 μl/well). Maintain cultures in C-DMEM at 37 °C in an atmosphere containing 5% CO_2/95% air. Change medium at 18–24 h and then every three days thereafter.

2.3.2 Adherence and shaking method

The protocol, given in detail below, is based on that described by Giulian and Baker for new-born rat brain microglia (13), but other groups use a similar technique. Mixed glia are plated into 75 cm² flasks and maintained *in vitro*. After seven days flasks are shaken to release loosely attached microglia into the medium whilst astrocytes remain attached. Microglia are then transferred to further flasks and allowed to adhere for 1–3 h. Gentle shaking of these flasks removes oligodendrocytes and the adherent microglia are removed with trypsin (in some laboratories, a rubber policeman is used to dislodge the microglia mechanically, usually after a shorter 15–30 min adherence step). The microglia can then be subjected to a second adherence step for 1–3 h, trypsinized again, and re-plated (*Protocol 3*).

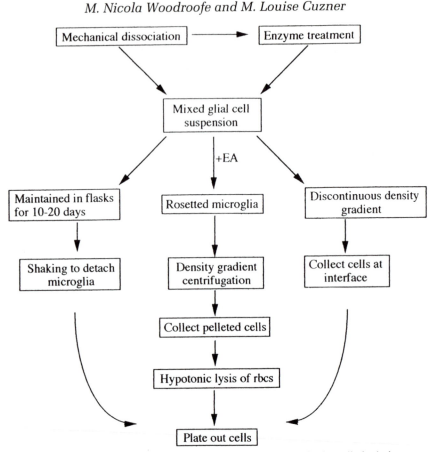

Figure 1. Schematic representation of the variety of methods of microglia isolation.

Protocol 3. Shaking and adherence method for isolation of microglia (13)

Equipment and reagents

- See *Protocol 1*
- 75 cm² Falcon tissue culture flasks (Gibco)
- Orbital shaker

Method

1. Follow *Protocol 2*, steps 1–6, up to the mixed glia suspension stage.
2. Plate mixed glia cell suspension in C-DMEM into a 75 cm² flask at a density of 8.5×10^5 cells/ml, 10 ml/flask.
3. Leave in incubator (5% CO_2/95% air, 37 °C) for seven to ten days, change the medium after three to four days.

4. Place flasks on an orbital shaker for 15–20 h (180 r.p.m.) at 37 °C.

5. Collect cells released into the supernatant, spin down and resuspend in C-DMEM, plate into fresh flasks at a density of 10^5 cells/ml, and adhere at 37 °C.

6. After 1–2 h, remove supernatant and any non-attached cells, and discard.

7. Maintain microglia *in vitro* in flasks or trypsinize with vigorous shaking (0.1% trypsin for 10 min) to remove microglia. Wash cells, plate out, and maintain as in *Protocol 2*.

8. Step 7 can be repeated to improve the purity of the preparation.

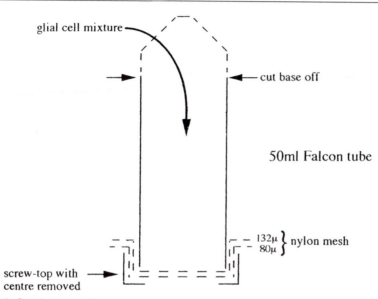

glial cell mixture

cut base off

50ml Falcon tube

132μ
80μ } nylon mesh

screw-top with
centre removed

Figure 2. Cut the base off a 50 ml Falcon tube and the centre out of its screw-top. Place one piece each of 132 μm and 80 μm porosity nylon mesh over the end of the tube and secure these using the cap as indicated. Methanol sterilize the 'sieve' before use. The mixture of glial cells can now be poured through the cut end of the tube.

2.3.3 Discontinuous density gradient

This method allows isolation of microglia from a mixed glia suspension without rosetting, by centrifugation on a discontinuous gradient of Percoll (5). The gradient consists of five steps starting with a density of 1.122 g/ml at the bottom of the tube, followed by 1.088 g/ml which contains the cell suspension, then 1.072 g/ml, 1.03 g/ml, and finally a layer of Hank's buffer. The interface between the 1.072 g/ml and 1.088 g/ml Percoll steps is harvested and contains the microglia.

2.4 Advantages and disadvantages of the methods

The major disadvantage of the adherence and shaking method is the length of time the cells are in culture prior to obtaining purified microglia (usually two to three weeks), and the question of whether the phenotypic and functional characteristics of the microglia has changed during this period. A criticism of the rosetting technique is that this procedure may activate the cells and thereby bias *in vitro* studies. However peritoneal macrophages which have been rosetted show little difference in functional properties when compared with non-rosetted macrophages (4). This method may also select a subpopulation of microglia expressing the Fc receptor (FcR), although there is widespread readily detectable FcR expression *in vivo* in both neonatal and adult mouse brain (14). The recovery of microglia by shaking methods is also selective on the basis of adhesion parameters, in some cases as little as 10% of the total microglia is recovered (13). The discontinuous gradient method (5) has no apparent disadvantages but has been little used by other laboratories; it may only be a matter of time before this method gains wider acceptance. Since microglia isolated from fetal and neonatal animals may not share identical properties (14) it is preferable to use cells isolated from the adult brain, when their role in pathological events in the adult animal is being investigated. Gradient techniques are particularly suitable for adult glial preparations, since the myelin in these bands at the interface and does not interfere with the microglia separation. Since microglia are phagocytic cells they become engorged with myelin if cultured in its presence (K. Mosley, unpublished data) and detach from the flasks. The adherence of microglia to flasks would be prevented by the presence of myelin when the adherence method is applied to adult tissue. Separation of myelin from the mixed glia before they are plated into flasks is therefore advantageous (6).

2.5 Cell yields

Few data are available on yields of microglia obtained by the various isolation methods. Guilian and Baker (13) recovered 10% of the initial non-specific esterase (NSE+) cells in the mixed glia suspension. 10^6 mixed glia were isolated from a ten-day-old mouse brain of which up to 10^5 would be microglia (15). The gradient separation methods give similar cell yields; by the discontinuous density gradient method 4×10^5 microglia were obtained from a three to four-week-old rat brain (5) and the yield of microglia following isolation by the rosetting method varies between 5–15×10^5 cells/g starting tissue, with neonatal rat brain giving higher yields than adult rat (4).

2.6 Culture media

Earle's balanced salt solution (EBSS) or Hank's balanced salt solution (HBSS) are generally used for the dissociation steps of the microglial isolation. Dulbecco's modified Eagle medium (DMEM) is preferred for maintaining microglia *in vitro*, generally supplemented with 10% fetal calf serum, 2 mM glutamine, and antibiotics (e.g. penicillin–streptomycin or gentamycin) (15). Eagles minimal essential medium (MEM) supplemented with insulin in addition to the above is also used (11). Microglia can be maintained in serum-free defined medium, e.g. N1 (16) or M1 (Gibco-BRL) (K. Mosley, unpublished data).

3. Cellular markers for microglia

The purity of the microglia preparations obtained by the isolation procedure is determined with microglia/macrophage-specific monoclonal antibodies or by functional markers. *Table 1* lists the monoclonal antibodies generally used, their specificities, and the supplier. In this laboratory immunocyto-chemical staining of microglia is performed using an avidin–biotin peroxidase method as described in *Protocol 4*. Functional markers of microglia which are not species-specific are also used to establish cell purity (*Table 1*), usually non-specific esterase (NSE) activity is measured however this is not always satisfactory. Adult microglia from human brain being NSE[-] *in vitro* (6) whereas human fetal microglia were NSE[+] (7). In this laboratory it has been observed that adult rat microglia are NSE[-] and new-born rat microglia are only weakly positive (*Figure 3*) when compared with blood monocytes maintained *in vitro* for the same period of time. An alternative functional marker commonly used is the phagocytic index which is discussed below (see 6(i)).

Table 1. Cell markers for microglia

Monoclonal antibody	Specificity	Supplier	Species	Reference
EBM/11	Cytoplasmic antigen	Dako	Human	17
Leu M5	CD11c	Becton Dickinson	Human	18
OX42	CR3	Serotec	Rat	19
ED1	97 kDa antigen	Serotec	Rat	20
MAC 1	CD11b, CD18	Boehringer Mann	Mouse	21
Functional markers for MG[a]				
Dil-ac-LDL		Molecular probes Inc.,		13
(acetylated low density lipoprotein with fluorescent label)		Oregon, USA.		
FcR, C3bR		Dako		4
Phagocytosis of latex beads		Polysciences Inc. Ltd.		22
Non-specific esterase (NSE)		Sigma kit		23
Lectins, e.g. Ricinius communis agglutinin and GS1-β4		Sigma		24–26

[a] These are not species-specific.

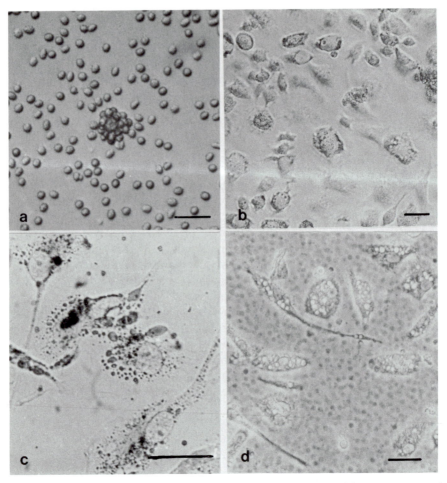

Figure 3. Microglia rosetted with opsonized red cells are separated from non-rosetted glial cells by Percoll density gradient centrifugation (a). Rat brain microglia maintained in serum-free medium (M1, Gibco) for 11 days, after being in C-DMEM for 4 days (b). NSE⁺ neonatal rat brain microglia in C-DMEM (c) and also after phagocytosis of EA which can be seen inside the microglia (d). Bar represents 25 μm.

Protocol 4. Immunocytochemical staining of microglia

Equipment and reagents

- Paraformaldehyde (BDH) 4% in PBS, prepare freshly by heating to 60 °C with stirring—filter through Whatman No.1 filter paper before use
- Antibodies (see *Table 1*)
- PBS/0.5% BSA
- Avidin–biotin peroxidase kit (ABC kit, Vector Laboratories)

- 3'3 Diaminobenzidine–HCl (Sigma) (25 mg/ml stock solution) (NB: DAB is carcinogenic; wear gloves when handling)
- H₂O₂ (30% v/v) (BDH)
- Mouse IgG1 Kappa (MOPC 21) myeloma protein (Sigma)

Method

1. Fix the cultures for 10 min in 4% paraformaldehyde at room temperature.

2. Further fix as appropriate for 2 min in either cold acetic acid/alcohol (5 : 95) (for glial fibrillary acidic protein, GFAP), ethanol (OX42), or acetone (ED1, EBM/11). Rinse in PBS three or four times.

3. Include control slides where the first antibody is substituted with myeloma protein of the same immunoglobulin subclass and concentration in all staining runs.

4. Remove the plastic walls of the chamber slide, leaving the gasket around each well intact to prevent the antibodies from mixing.

5. Add 50 μl of diluted antibody or control (in PBS/0.5% BSA) to each well and maintain in a humid box for 1 h at room temperature.

6. Rinse the slide three times in PBS and drain the excess PBS from the wells.

7. Slides are immunostained by the avidin–biotin peroxidase method (ABC).

8. Add 50 μl of biotinylated anti-mouse antibody (diluted 1 : 200 in PBS to each well). Incubate for 30 min at room temperature.

9. Repeat step 6 and then add 50 μl of the preformed avidin–biotin peroxidase complex and incubate for 45 min.

10. Repeat step 6. Remove the rubber gasket from the slide using forceps.

11. Visualize the bound antibody by immersing the slide in the substrate which consists of 8 ml of stock DAB solution, 400 ml PBS, and 167 μl H_2O_2 (30% v/v). (Final concentrations are 0.5 mg/ml DAB, 0.01% H_2O_2.) After 2–3 min, check the staining intensity and either rinse in H_2O or replace in substrate solution to increase the intensity of staining.

    NB: DAB is carcinogenic, wear gloves at this stage.

12. Add one drop of PBS/glycerol (50 : 50) and place a coverslip over the slide, seal with nail varnish, and view.

4. Microglial morphology

The *in vivo* amoeboid, bipolar rod-shaped, and ramified morphological types have been described in cultured microglia (*Figure 3*). The ramified cells in culture closely resemble the adult cell morphology *in vivo*, whereas amoeboid cells are similar to microglia in the neonate. In the presence of lipopolysaccharide (LPS), colony stimulating factor (CSF)-1, or LPS-stimulated astrocyte supernatant microglia undergo reversible morphological transformations *in vitro*, adopting respectively amoeboid, rod-shaped, and ramified morphologies (27).

Acknowledgements

This work was supported by the Brain Research Trust and the Multiple Sclerosis Society of Great Britain. The authors would like to thank Dr Jane Loughlin, Karen Mosley, and Dr Gillian Hayes for their contributions, and Jenny Damji for secretarial assistance.

References

1. Theele, D. P. and Streit, W. J. (1993). *GLIA*, **7**, 5.
2. Lawson, L. J., Perry, V. H., Dri, P., and Gordon, S. (1990). *Neuroscience*, **39**, 151.
3. McCarthy, K. D. and de Vellis, J. (1980). *J. Cell Biol.*, **85**, 890.
4. Hayes, G. M., Woodroofe, M. N., and Cuzner, M. L. (1988). *J. Neuroimmunol.*, **19**, 177.
5. Sedgwick, J. D., Schwender, S., Imrich, H., Dorries, R., Butcher, G. W., and Meulen, V. T. (1991). *Proc. Natl. Acad. Sci. USA*, **88**, 7438.
6. Williams, K., Bar-Or, A., Ulvestad, E., Olivier, A., Antel, J. P., and Yong, V. W. (1992). *J. Neuropathol. Exp. Neurol.*, **51**, 538.
7. Peudenier, S., Hery, C., Montagnier, L., and Tardieu, M. (1991). *Ann. Neurol.*, **29**, 152.
8. Graeber, M. B., Banati, R. B., Streit, W. J., and Kreutzberg, G. W. (1989). *Neurosci. Lett.*, **103**, 241.
9. Matsumoto, Y., Ohmori, K., and Fujiwara, M. (1992). *Immunology*, **76**, 209.
10. Suzumura, A., Mezitis, S. G. E., Gonatas, N. K., and Silberberg, D. H. (1987). *J. Neuroimmunol.*, **15**, 263.
11. Chao, C. C., Molitor, T. W., Shaskan, E. G., and Peterson, P. K. (1992). *J. Immunol.*, **149**, 2736.
12. Newcombe, J., Meeson, A., and Cuzner, M. L. (1988). *Neuropathol. Appl. Neurobiol.*, **14**, 453.
13. Giulian, D. and Baker, T. J. (1986). *J. Neurosci.*, **6**, 2163.
14. Perry, V. H. and Gordon, S. (1991). *Int. Rev. Cytol.*, **125**, 203.
15. Moore, S. C., McCormack, J. M., Armendariz, E., Gatewood, J., and Walker, W. S. (1992). *J. Neuroimmunol.*, **41**, 203.
16. Bottenstein, J. E. and Sato, G. H. (1979). *Proc. Natl. Acad. Sci. USA*, **76**, 514.
17. Esiri, M. M. and McGee, J. O. D. (1986). *J. Clin. Pathol.*, **39**, 615.
18. Lanier, L. L., Amaout, M. A., Schwarting, R., Warner, N. L., and Ross, G. D. (1985). *Eur. J. Immunol.*, **15**, 713.
19. Robinson, A. P., White, T. M., and Mason, D. W. (1986). *Immunology*, **57**, 239.
20. Dijkstra, C. D., Dopp, E. A., Joling, P., and Kraal, G. (1985). *Immunology*, **54**, 589.
21. Springer, T. A. and Ho, M. K. (1982). In *Hybridomas in Cancer Diagnosis and Treatment*. (ed. M. S. Mitchell and H. F. Oettagen), pp. 35–46. Raven Press, New York.

22. Dubois, J. H., Hammond-Tooke, G. D., and Cuzner, M. L. (1985). *Int. J. Dev. Neurosci.*, **3,** 531.
23. Ling, E. A. (1981). *Adv. Cell. Neurobiol.*, **2,** 33.
24. Mannoji, H., Yeger, H., and Becker, L. E. (1986). *Acta Neuropathol.*, **71,** 341.
25. Colton, C. A., Abel, C., Patchett, J., Keri, J., and Yao, J. B. (1992). *J. Histochem. Cytochem.*, **40,** 505.
26. Yao, J. B., Keri, J. E., Taffs, R. E., and Colton, C. A. (1992). *Brain Res.*, **591,** 88.
27. Suzumura, A., Marunouchi, T., and Yamamoto, H. (1991). *Brain Res.*, **545,** 301.

10

Brain endothelium

DAVID MALE

1. Introduction

The endothelium of the CNS, including that of the retina is quite distinct from endothelium in other tissues. It has continuous tight junctions, low numbers of vesicles, and a variety of characteristic surface molecules (1). In addition, it lacks many of the molecules found on large vessel or microvessel endothelia from outside the brain. *In vivo* the electrical resistance across CNS endothelium is in excess of 2000 Ohms/cm^2, although the best *in vitro* cultures only approach 500 Ohms/cm^2 (2). The factors which control the expression of this distinctive phenotype are not known, but there may be an astrocytic influence via cytokines (3). *In vitro*, primary cultures of brain endothelium have been obtained from rat, mouse, bovine, chick, and human brain. Some of the primary cultures have been propagated for extended periods (4), however we have found that many of the distinctive features of rat CNS endothelium are lost after a number of passages.

This chapter describes a method for the isolation of CNS capillary endothelium from rat, and its propagation *in vitro* in primary culture. The method was originally developed by Dr C. C. W. Hughes (5), based on previously described techniques (6,7). We have used these cultures extensively for immunological studies on lymphocyte migration across CNS endothelium, and for the analysis of surface molecule expression and response to cytokines. The final section refers to some of the methods used to isolate endothelium from other species.

2. Isolation of capillary fragments

2.1 General considerations

The method described uses two rats and provides sufficient endothelium to cover a 96-well microtitre plate or two small tissue culture flasks (25 cm^2). Endothelium can be isolated from any strain, however the growth rates and degree of contamination vary between strains. We have found Lewis rats aged two to three months to be most satisfactory, but other inbred or outbred strains of this age can also be used. The method uses a first digestion to separate capillaries from other CNS components, followed by a BSA gradient to isolate the capillaries. Then the capillaries undergo a second digestion to separate contaminating cells, and the endothelium is isolated on a Percoll gradient.

Protocol 1. Isolation of rat brain capillary endothelium

Equipment and reagents

All reagents should be sterile filtered.

- Sterile squares of gauze, Petri dish, and beakers
- Sterile dissecting instruments, including scalpel, fine bent forceps, and jeweller's forceps
- Medium-1: Ca^{2+}/Mg^{2+}-free Hank's balanced salt solution containing 10 mM Hepes, 100 U/ml penicillin, and 100 µg/ml streptomycin, adjusted to pH 7.4 and sterile filtered

- 25 ml of 250 mg/ml bovine serum albumin (BSA) in medium-1
- 25 ml aliquots of 1 mg/ml collagenase/dispase (Boehringer) in medium-1
- 250 µl aliquots of 1 mg/ml DNase (Sigma, D-4263) in medium-1
- 25 µl aliquots of tosyl lysyl cholecystokinine (TLCK; Sigma) at 0.147 mg/ml in distilled water

(a) Immediately before starting make up working medium by oxygenating 125 ml of medium-1 for 10 min (bubble O_2 through a sterile Pasteur pipette). Then add 2.5 ml of 250 mg/ml BSA, to a final concentration of 5 mg/ml BSA. This is general purpose medium (medium-P) which is kept on ice for use throughout the preparation.

(b) A Percoll gradient is needed for separation of the capillary component cells (step 16). This is prepared just before use from 7 ml of isotonic sterile 50% Percoll (Sigma), in a tube which may be sterilized with 70% ethanol, and which is then rinsed with medium-P, to minimize sticking of capillaries to the sides. The gradient is made by centrifuging the 50% Percoll for 1 h at 25 000 *g* at 10 °C.

Method

1. Kill the rat, remove the brain, and transfer to medium-P on ice.

2. Dissect on a gauze square dampened with medium-P on a Petri dish. (See *Figure 1*, for steps 2–4 of the dissection.) Remove the cerebellum and take one cerebral hemisphere.

3. Using jeweller's forceps and starting at the circle of Willis, remove the meninges. Clean off any residual meninges by rolling the hemisphere on dry sterile gauze.

4. Using curved forceps, remove the midbrain, and as much of the white matter as is reasonably accessible. This leaves grey matter of the cerebral cortex.

5. Place the cortex in 20 ml of medium-P on ice and chop with a scalpel into small cubes of 1–2 mm².

6. Repeat for the second hemisphere.

7. Repeat for the second rat.

8. Spin down the fragments (300 *g*, 5 min) and resuspend in 20 ml of collagenase/dispase, with the addition of 200 μl DNase and 20 μl TLCK. Incubate for 1 h at 37 °C (first digestion).

9. The digest should be thoroughly broken up by repeated aspiration through sterile Pasteur pipettes. Start with a normal Pasteur, and then use Pasteurs with a reduced bore size (produced by flaming the end).

10. Spin down the digest (300 *g*, 5 min) and remove the supernatant.

11. Add 20 ml of 250 mg/ml BSA solution, and completely redistribute the digest in the BSA solution by repeated aspiration through a fine-bore Pasteur pipette.

12. Centrifuge the tube at 1000 *g* for 20 min. Carefully tilt and rotate the tube and pour off the myelin plug and the BSA solution. The pellet contains the capillaries (*Figure 2a*).

13. Transfer to a clean tube in 10 ml of medium-P.

14. Spin down the capillary fragments, and resuspend in 5 ml of collage-nase/dispase with 50 μl DNase and 5 μl of TLCK. Incubate for 3 h at 37 °C (second digestion). Oxygenation of the digest (bubbling for 2 min) is beneficial but not essential.

15. Spin down the digest and resuspend in 1 ml of medium-P.

16. Layer the digest on to the Percoll gradient, and centrifuge at 1000 *g* for 10 min. Remove the capillary fragments from the central zone of the gradient (*Figure 2b*), and resuspend in 10 ml of medium-P.

17. Spin down and wash twice in medium-P, before resuspending in 10–15 ml of growth medium for plating out. Use 150 μl of cell suspension per microtitre well (96-well plate) or 5 ml of suspension for a small flask.

3. Growth conditions

3.1 Substrata

Unlike most other endothelia, CNS endothelium has an absolute require-ment for an extracellular matrix to attach to and to promote outgrowth. Flasks should be coated with 0.3 mg/ml sterile type-1 collagen for 30 min. This is then removed and the collagen fixed by transferring to a box contain-ing NH_3 vapour for a further 30 min. This can be done by placing a plug of cotton wool soaked in a few drops of 880 ammonia solution in a sandwich box together with the tissue culture plate or flask. The flasks are then rinsed three times with BSS before the endothelial cells are put in.

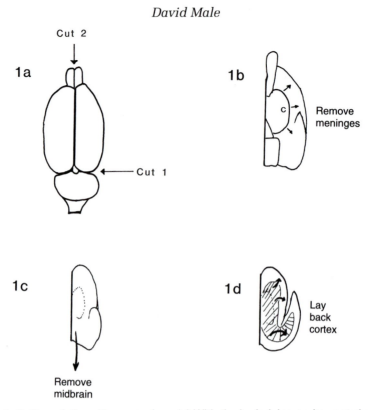

Figure 1. Outline of dissection procedure. (a) With the brain lying on its ventral surface, remove cerebellum (cut 1) and separate the two halves of the brain (cut 2). (b) With the half brain on its dorsal surface, starting at the Circle of Willis (c) use jeweller's forceps to remove meninges as arrowed, around to the dorsal midline. Remove residual fragments by rolling on dry guaze. (c) With the brain on its dorsal surface, using dental forceps, remove the midbrain, any remaining hindbrain, and olfactory bulbs. (d) Lay back the temporal cortex as arrowed, exposing white matter underlying the cortex. Using curved forceps, pick off white matter from the hatched area.

3.2 Growth media and conditions

Cells are grown in Ham's F-10 medium, containing 20% plasma-derived serum, 2 mM glutamine, 100 µg/ml streptomycin, 100 U/ml penicillin, 40 µg/ml heparin, 75 µg/ml endothelial cell growth supplement (ECGS; Sigma, E-2759), and 5 µg/ml ascorbic acid. It is possible to use gentamycin (40 µg/ml) in the cultures, but amphotericin-B (fungizone) at the concentrations usually used in tissue culture (25 µg/ml) is toxic.

The medium shoud be completely replaced two days after plating out, and thereafter every three days. Initially the cells appear as small capillary trees containing 20–200 cells. After 24 hours these have rolled up into clumps of cells. By 48 hours the endothelial cells start to spread across the plate/flask.

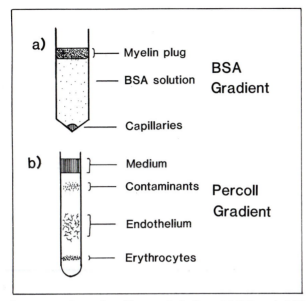

Figure 2. Gradient separations of capillary endothelium. (a) 250 mg/ml BSA used to separate capillaries from other CNS components. (b) 50% Isotonic Percoll gradient, used to separate endothelial cells from other cells associated with capillaries.

Cell division occurs maximally from days two to six and the cells form confluent monolayers six to ten days after plating out (*Figure 3*).

The particular formulation of the medium uses plasma-derived serum since PDGF present in, for example, fetal calf serum, favours the growth of contaminating smooth muscle cells or fibroblasts (8). ECGS contains acidic fibroblast growth factor (aFGF), and heparin acts as a growth cofactor (9). Platelet-derived endothelial cell growth factor (not to be confused with PDGF) may also be used to promote division (10).

Originally plasma-derived serum was difficult to obtain, but it is now commercially available (Advanced Protein Products). The following method may be used to prepare it, should commercial batches be unsatisfactory.

Protocol 2. Preparation of plasma-derived serum

1. Ensure that plastic containers are used throughout the preparation, until the platelets have been separated. Also use plastic pipettes, etc.

2. Make up trisodium citrate solution at 3.8 g/100 ml. Collect bovine blood into 10% citrate on ice, giving a final concentration of 0.38 g citrate/100 ml.

3. Spin at 1200 g for 18 min to remove red cells.

Protocol 2. *Continued*

4. Take the plasma and centrifuge at 24000 *g* for 20 min at 4 °C to remove platelets.

5. Recalcify the plasma by adding 1 M CaCl₂ to a final concentration of 20 mM. Leave overnight to clot.

6. Remove fibrin by spinning at 4 °C for 30 min at 24000 *g*.

7. Dialyse against Hepes/saline (10 mM Hepes/0.9% NaCl, pH 7.2).

8. To remove residual PDGF, add 10% (v/v) CM–Sephadex in Hepes/saline. Leave for 30 min and spin or filter out the beads.

9. Heat inactivate the serum (56 °C, 30 min).

10. Sterile filter and store at –20 °C.

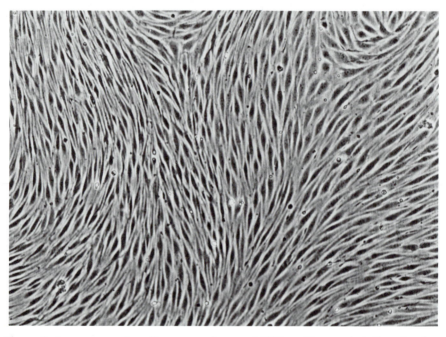

Figure 3. Appearance of confluent monolayers of CNS capillary endothelium *in vitro*, viewed by phase-contrast light microscopy. Unlike large vessel endothelium in culture, these cells retain the elongated form seen *in vivo*.

3.3 Passaging the cells

We have found that the specific phenotype of brain endothelial cells cultured in this way decays with repeated passages of the cells. For some purposes however it is desirable to seed new cultures from the primary culture. To do this, the endothelium should be rinsed in Ca²⁺/Mg²⁺-free BSS, and digested for 5 min in a minimum volume of 0.5 mg/ml trypsin. Once the cells have detached in small groups, the trypsin should be neutralized by the addition of an equal volume of fetal calf serum, then spun down, washed twice in BSS, and resuspended in growth medium, before plating out on to new wells/flasks. It is essential that the new wells are coated with collagen as above.

The method above generates endothelial cell cultures with a high level of purity. Should it be necessary to improve the purity, various measures can be used (*Protocol 3*).

Protocol 3. Removal of contaminating cells

1. Wash the endothelium with cold Ca^{2+}/Mg^{2+}-free BSS at the time of the first medium exchange (day two). This preferentially detaches contaminants.

2. Pericytes may be killed by treatment with anti-Thy-1 antibody and complement (11).

3. Culturing the cells in medium containing D-valine, which prevents the growth of fibroblasts, but not endothelium (12).

It should be emphasized that these steps should not normally be necessary. They may be included if contamination by non-endothelial cells is high, as determined by phenotyping of the cultures.

4. Phenotyping

Brain endothelial cell monolayers appear as continuous swirling sheets of flat bipolar cells, which are only readily visible using phase-contrast, inverted microscopy. They are fully contact inhibited. Cultures obtained by the method described should be greater than 95% pure endothelium. The principal contaminating cells are pericytes, smooth muscle, and fibroblasts. These cells are all associated with vessels. Pericytes appear as occasional irregular cells overlying the monolayer, which have not grown out from the original capillary fragment. They express the enzymes γ-glutamyl transferase and cyclic GMP-dependent protein kinase (13). Smooth muscle cells grow in strands, which may overlie the endothelial cells. They are less flattened than the endothelium. Fibroblasts are difficult to distinguish from brain endothelium visually, but are usually irregular and do not make edge contact with the endothelial cells.

Phenotyping of the cells by, for example, immunofluorescence is one way to be certain of the identity of the cells isolated (14). *Table 1* lists a number of useful markers which may be used to confirm the identity of rat brain endothelium. Brain endothelium expresses many of the markers present on

Table 1. Brain endothelial cell phenotype discrimination

Marker	Comment
von Willebrand Factor	Present on all endothelial cells
Angiotensin converting enzyme (ACE)	Present on all endothelia
Transferrin receptor (15)	Expressed on CNS endothelium, but not non-CNS endothelium
OX-45 and OX-46 (16)	Antibodies identify all rat endothelia
ZO-1 (17)	Antibody identifies tight junctions
p-Glycoprotein (18)	Product of multidrug resistance gene expressed on CNS endothelium
γ-Glutamyl transferase	Identifies contaminating pericytes
cGMP-dependent protein kinase (19)	Identifies pericytes and smooth muscle

other endothelia, but also has continuous tight junctions, and some specialized transport systems. In addition to those markers listed in *Table 1*, the acetylated LDL-receptor expression is frequently used to identify rat CNS endothelium however at least one report indicates that both the LDL-receptor and the acetylated LDL-receptor are absent from bovine brain capillaries (20).

If available, transmission electron microscopy can be used to show tight junctions. Alternatively, antibodies may be used to identify junction components. The lectin BSB4 (21) has also been used to identify endothelium, although immunofluorescent staining is not usually strong. Ulex Europaeus lectin binds to the luminal surface of endothelium (22). Surface molecules on brain endothelium may also be readily quantitated using a cell surface enzyme immunoassay (23).

5. Problems

The principal problems which may arise with the technique described are low yield, poor attachment of the capillary fragments, slow cell growth, or fast growth of contaminating cells.

The yield of a preparation can be increased by resuspending the myelin plug in the BSA for a second time and repeating the centrifugation (*Protocol 1*, steps 11–13). This produces a second pellet of capillary fragments.

Poor attachment is usually caused by an incomplete second digest, or failure to fix the collagen on the flask properly.

The principal variable in the preparation is the plasma-derived serum (PDS). Poor endothelial cell growth, or overgrowth of contaminants is often due to a bad batch of PDS. Ensure that the PDS is correctly prepared, and fully dialysed after the preparation. Low levels of contamination by non-endothelial cells may be reduced by rinsing the attached cells at their first feed (day two) with cold Ca^{2+}/Mg^{2+}-free balanced salt solution. This preferentially detaches contaminant cells.

For enhancing the electrical resistance of the monolayers, many groups have used astrocyte-conditioned medium (24) or enhancers of cyclic AMP, including forskolin. The mechanisms by which these supplements act has not been defined.

6. CNS endothelium from other species

The technique described above has been adapted to produce mouse CNS endothelium, and should be of general utility. From man and other species, particularly older individuals, there is an increasing risk of contamination with fibroblasts. Different methods of confirmed value have been described for human (25) and bovine CNS endothelium (26,27). The antibody PAL-E is useful for the identification of human endothelia, although it does not bind to rat endothelia (28).

References

1. Bradbury, M. W. B. (ed). (1992). *Physiology and pharmacology of the blood brain barrier. Handbook of experimental pharmacology*, Vol. 103. Springer-Verlag.
2. Greenwood, J. (1991). *Ann. N. Y. Acad. Sci.*, **633,** 426.
3. Arthur, R. E., Shivers, R. R., and Bowman, P. D. (1987). *Dev. Brain Res.*, **36,** 155.
4. Spatz, M. and Mrsulja, B. B. (1982). *Brain Res.*, **191,** 577.
5. Hughes, C. C. W. and Lantos, P. L. (1986). *Neurosci. Lett.*, **68,** 100.
6. Goldstein, G. W., Betz, A. L., and Bowman, P. D. (1984). *Fed. Proc.*, **43,** 191.
7. Audus, K. L. and Borchardt, R. T. (1986). *Pharm. Res.*, **3,** 81.
8. Williams, L. T. (1989). *Science*, **243,** 1564.
9. Hiroyoshi, H. and McKeehan, W. L. (1984). *Proc. Natl. Acad. Sci. USA*, **81,** 6413.
10. Miyazoni, K. and Heldin, C. H. (1989). *Biochemistry*, **28,** 1704.
11. Risau, W., Engelhardt, B., and Wekerle, H. (1990). *J. Cell Biol.*, **110,** 1757.
12. Picciano, P. T., Johnson, B., Walenga, R. W., Donovan, M., Borman, B. J., Douglas, H. J., *et al.* (1984). *Exp. Cell Res.*, **151,** 134.
13. Rutenberg, A. M., Kim, H., Fischbein, J. W., Hanker, J. S., Wasserkrug, H. L., and Seligman, A. M. (1969). *J. Histochem. Cytochem.*, **17,** 517.
14. Abbott, N. J., Hughes, C. C., Revest, P. A. and Greenwood, J. (1992). *J. Cell Sci.*, **103,** 23.
15. Jefferies, W. A., Brandon, M. R., Hunt, S. V., Williams, A. F., Gatter, K. C., and Mason, D. Y. (1984). *Nature*, **312,** 162.
16. Arvieux, J., Willis, A. C., and Williams, A. F. (1986). *Mol. Immunol.*, **23,** 983.
17. Watson, P. M., Anderson, J. M., Voultallie, C. M., and Doctrow, S. R. (1991). *Neurosci. Lett.*, **6,** 10.
18. Cordon-Cardo, C., O'Brien, J. P., Casals, D., Rittman-Grauer, L., Biedler, J. L., Melamed, M. R., *et al.* (1989). *Proc. Natl. Acad. Sci. USA*, **86,** 695.
19. Joyce, N. C., DeCamilli, P., and Boyles, J. (1984). *Microvasc. Res.*, **28,** 206.

David Male

20. Gaffney, J., West, D., Arnold, F., Saltar, A., and Kumar, S. (1985). *J. Cell Sci.*, **79,** 317.
21. Tontsch, U. and Bauer, H. C. (1989). *Microvasc. Res.*, **37,** 148.
22. Vorbrodt, A. W., Dobrogowska, D. H., Lossinsky, A. S., and Wisniewski, H. M. (1986). *J. Histochem. Cytochem.*, **34,** 251.
23. Male, D. K., Pryce, G., and Hughes, C. C. W. (1987). *Immunology*, **60,** 453.
24. Raub, T., Kuentzel, S. L., and Sawada, G. A. (1992). *Exp. Cell Res.*, **199,** 330.
25. Dorovini-Zis, K., Prameya, R., and Bowman, P. (1991). *Lab. Invest.*, **64,** 425.
26. Bowman, P. D., Ennis, S. R., Rarey, K. E., Betz, A. L., and Goldstein, G. W. (1983). *Ann. Neurol.*, **14,** 396.
27. Rubin, L. L., Hall, D. E., Porter, S., Barbu, K., Cannon, C., Horner, H. C., *et al.* (1991). *J. Cell Biol.*, **115,** 1725.
28. Schlingemann, R. O., Dingjun, G. M., Emeis, J. J., Blok, J., Warnaar, S., and Ruiter, D. (1985). *Lab. Invest.*, **52,** 71.

III. PNS neurons and glia

Neural crest cells: strategies to generate lineage diversification *in vitro*

JEAN-LOUP DUBAND, MURIEL DELANNET, and
FREDERIQUE MONIER

1. Introduction

The neural crest is both a curiosity and a spectacular invention of vertebrates. It consists of a population of precursor cells endowed with striking migratory properties and possessing an extraordinary range of potentialities. The neural crest develops all along the embryonic axis, in the neural folds, at the boundary between the neural plate and the superficial ectoderm. However, neural crest cells do not remain at their site of origin after appearance. At a precise stage of embryonic development, e.g. soon after neural tube closure in birds, they venture out of the neural epithelium and disperse within the embryo along defined migratory pathways. After migration, neural crest cells settle in various regions of the embryo to generate a wide spectrum of derivatives ranging from cells that are truly neural (i.e. neurons of the peripheral nervous system) to others that are essentially mesodermal (1,2) (*Table 1*).

The neural crest is regionalized such that cells originating from different axial levels undergo migration at different developmental stages, follow distinct migratory pathway, and produce defined subsets of derivatives. Roughly, the development of the neural crest accompanies the rostro-caudal development of the embryo and follows the wave of segmentation of the paraxial mesoderm into the somites. Thus, four major regions can be identified in birds and mammals and have been designated as cranial, vagal, truncal, and lumbosacral (*Figure 1*). The cranial level corresponds to the forebrain, midbrain, and anterior hindbrain. Cranial neural crest cells migrate laterally under the ectoderm to reach the ventral regions of the head where cells contribute to connective tissues and skeleton of the face (the so-called mesectoderm or ectomesenchyme) and to the ciliary and some cranial sensory ganglia. The vagal region corresponds to the posterior hindbrain up to the seventh somite, the term vagal deriving from the vagus nerve which

Table 1. Neural crest derivatives

Neuronal cells
Autonomic ganglia (sympathetic, enteric, and ciliary)
Sensory ganglia
   All neurons of the spinal dorsal root ganglia
   Some neurons of the trigeminal (nerve V, trigeminal), geniculate (nerve VII, facial),
   superior (nerve IX, glossopharyngeal), and jugulare (nerve X, vagus) ganglia

Supporting cells of the nervous system
Schwann cells
Glial and satellite cells of the spinal sensory and autonomic ganglia
Glial and satellite cells of the cranial sensory ganglia: trigeminal (V), geniculate (VII),
acoustic (VIII), superior-petrosal (IX), jugulare-nodose (X) ganglia

Pigment cells
Melanocytes of dermis, mesenteries, internal organs, epidermis, etc., and melanophores
of the iris, but *not* the pigment cells of the retina

Endocrine and paraendocrine cells
Adrenomedullary cells and other adrenergic paraganglia
Calcitonin-producing cells in the ultimobranchial body
Types I and II cells of the carotid body

Ectomesenchyme (or mesectoderm)
Dermis of the face and ventral part of the neck
Connective tissues of the buccal and pharyngeal glands (salivary gland, thyroid,
parathyroid) and of the thymus
Fibroblasts and endothelium of the cornea
Musculoconnective wall of the large arteries derived from the aortic arches
Muscles: jaw opening and closing m., ocular m., tongue m., etc.
Bones and cartilage of the facial and hypobranchial skeleton and of the skull vault

originates from this region. At this level, neural crest cells follow both a lateral pathway like cranial neural crest cells, to provide chiefly mesectodermal tissues and cranial sensory ganglia and a ventral route leading them to the gut where they give rise to the enteric nervous system. In the trunk region (from the 8th somite to the 28th somite), neural crest cells migrate essentially along a ventral route and differentiate into the spinal sensory ganglia, the sympathetic chain and the adrenal medulla. In the lumbosacral region (from the 29th somite to the caudal end of the animal), although the migratory pathways of neural crest cells are not precisely determined, it is clear that they contribute, like their vagal counterparts, to the enteric nervous system, as well as to spinal and sympathetic ganglia.

The diversity of cell types derived from the neural crest makes this cell population an attractive system for investigating the processes of cell commitment and lineage diversification in vertebrates, and more specifically in the nervous system. In this respect, because of the analogies the neural crest

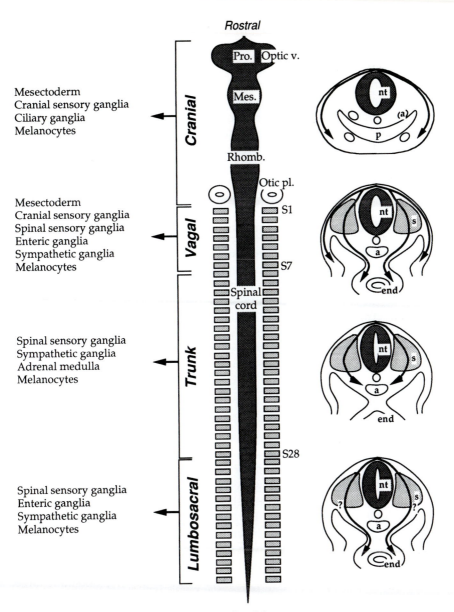

Rostral

Mesectoderm
Cranial sensory ganglia
Ciliary ganglia
Melanocytes

Cranial

Mesectoderm
Cranial sensory ganglia
Spinal sensory ganglia
Enteric ganglia
Sympathetic ganglia
Melanocytes

Vagal

Spinal sensory ganglia
Sympathetic ganglia
Adrenal medulla
Melanocytes

Trunk

Spinal sensory ganglia
Enteric ganglia
Sympathetic ganglia
Melanocytes

Lumbosacral

Pro. Optic v.

Mes.

Rhomb.

Otic pl.

S1

S7

Spinal cord

S28

Caudal

Figure 1. Schematic representation of the neural axis of an embryo showing the different portions of the central nervous system, i.e. prosencephalon (Pro.), mesencephalon (Mes.), rhombencephalon (Rhomb.) and spinal cord, the otic placodes (Otic pl.), the optic vesicles (Optic v.), the paravertebral mesoderm (somites S1...), and the corresponding neural crest regions: cranial, vagal, trunk, and lumbosacral. On the left are indicated the most representative derivatives of the neural crest populations originating from each region and, on the right, the principal migration routes of neural crest cells for each level are drawn schematically. Abbreviations: a, aorta; end, endoderm; g, gut; nt, neural tube; p, pharynx; s, somite.

135

system offers with haemopoietic cells, the term neuropoiesis has been proposed recently to account for the diverse range of neural cell types generated from this structure (3). On the other hand, due to its unique migratory properties, the neural crest provides an appropriate system for examining the mechanisms underlying cell locomotion. Finally, further interest of the neural crest system is that cells can be isolated from the embryo and grown in culture under conditions which mimic the different morphogenetic events that accompany the development of this structure *in vivo*, i.e. separation from the neural tube, migration, and differentiation.

2. Primary culture of neural crest cells

Although neural crest cells theoretically can be obtained from all axial levels, they are typically collected from the cranial and trunk regions. It should be kept in mind, however, that cranial and trunk neural crest cells cannot be isolated from the same developmental stage because the process of separation from the neural tube occurs gradually in a rostro-caudal sequence. *Table 2* shows the stages of development at which neural crest cells undergo migration at each axial level in the avian embryo and the corresponding optimal stages at which the embryos have to be collected for neural crest cell culture.

2.1 Truncal neural crest

2.1.1 Avian

Truncal neural crest cells are most commonly obtained from Japanese quails although they can also be obtained from White Leghorn chicks. Indeed, the timing of embryonic development in both species is very similar during the first four days of incubation. However, the quail embryo is usually preferred to the chick because, in the latter species, melanocytes are not pigmented and, consequently, neural crest differentiation cannot be followed as easily.

In the trunk, and also in the vagal and lumbosacral regions, migrating neural crest cells cannot be excised easily in large quantities and free of contaminating tissues because they are scattered in the sclerotome along the neural tube. Therefore, alternative approaches have to be developed for obtaining large,

---

Table 2. Timetable of neural crest cell migration

Embryonic level	Timing of separation[a]	Optimal stage for culture
Cranial	6–15 somites	10 somites (36 hours)
Vagal	10–18 somites	10 somites (36 hours)
Truncal	15–35 somites	20–28 somites (60 hours)

[a] The timing of separation corresponds to when neural crest cells are seen detaching from the neural epithelium.

---

homogeneous populations of neural crest cells. The easiest and most commonly used methodology was originally designed by Cohen (4). It utilizes the neural tube as a source of neural crest cells and is based on both the intrinsic migratory properties of neural crest cells and the fact that emigration occurs along a rostro-caudal gradient. The principle is to remove neural tubes from caudal regions of the trunk where it is known that neural crest cell migration at the stage considered has not yet begun and to explant them in culture. Although, in culture, cell dispersion occurs from explants of virtually any embryonic tissue, this process lasts several days and one might anticipate that neural crest cells, by virtue of their remarkable migratory potential, leave the explant earlier. Indeed, under appropriate conditions that facilitate the rapid attachment of the neural tube explant to the bottom of the dish, a number of cells separate within one to two hours and migrate. After 12–24 h of culture, these cells form an outgrowth of about 2000 to 3000 cells entirely surrounding the neural tube explant. All mesenchymal cells derived from the neural tube are neural crest cells (with the possible exception of a few cells situated at the cut ends of the neural tube explant), as demonstrated by expression of specific markers, including HNK-1 (5,6) and the ability of most cells to differentiate into neural crest-specific derivatives, such as melanocytes (4). In addition, the neural tube itself remains intact over the duration of culture and can be easily removed from the bottom of the dish, leaving behind a pure population of neural crest cells.

In order to obtain large outgrowths of neural crest cells, several conditions have to be fulfilled:

1. First, the stage of development of the embryo has to be chosen precisely and carefully. As indicated in *Table 2*, embryos should be in the stage range of 20–28 somite pairs, corresponding to approx. 60 h of incubation.

2. Secondly, the axial level from which the neural tube is explanted has to be defined appropriately. *Figures 2* and *3* illustrate the influence of the axial level of origin of the neural tube on the timing and nature of the neural crest outgrowth and on the morphology of individual cells. The optimal region for trunk neural crest culture corresponds to the six or seven last-formed somites and is indicated by region A in *Figure 2–1*. Explants corresponding to this region generally yield large outgrowths of several hundred cells up to 3000 cells within 12–18 h of culture. In addition, cells exhibit a well spread morphology with several processes per cell (*Figure 3A*). In contrast, if portions of neural tube are taken from more caudal levels, i.e. adjacent to the unsegmented mesoderm (region B in *Figure 2–1*), neural crest cells are not mature enough to commence emigration and the neural tube does not form a compact epithelium. Consequently, such neural tube explants tend to disaggregate in culture, and only a limited number of neural crest cells are able to migrate away from them. The few cells that are able to escape from the neural tube form a dense population of highly cohesive, flattened cells that show

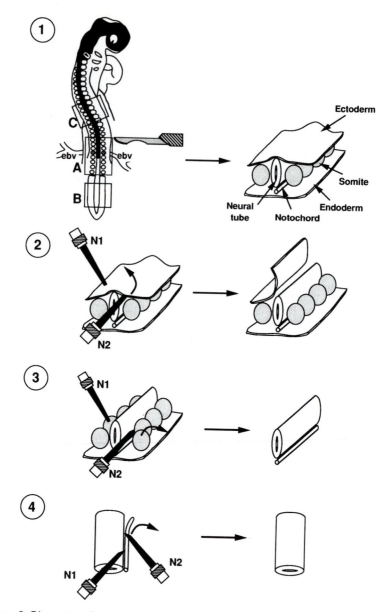

Figure 2. Diagrammatic sequence to dissect truncal neural tube explants from 2.5-day-old avian embryos. (1) Dissection of the trunk portions with a scalpel. The portion of the neural tube in black corresponds to the axial levels at which neural crest cell migration has started. The 21st pair of somites where the extraembryonic blood vessels (ebv) enter the embryo proper is shaded. (2) Removal of the ectoderm with needles. One of the needles (N1) maintains the explant in place while the other (N2) is introduced under the ectoderm and removes the ectoderm. (3) Removal of the somites. As for the previous step, needle N1 maintains the explant in place while needle N2 gently separates the somites from the neural tube. (4) Removal of the notochord. While needle N1 is placed in between the notochord and the neural tube, needle N2 gradually separates both tissue.

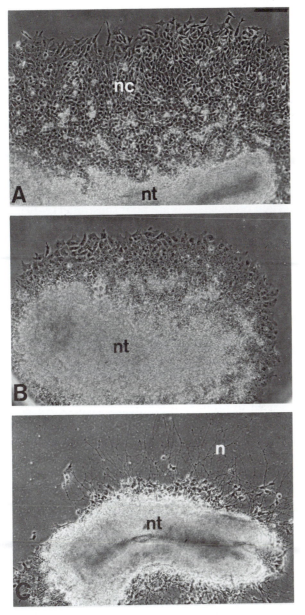

Figure 3. Morphology of neural crest outgrowths and of neural tube explants obtained from the three axial levels shown in *Figure 2–1* after 18 hours in culture. Neural tubes obtained from regions corresponding to the last formed somites (A) remain in shape and produce numerous neural crest cells, in contrast to neural tubes from either more caudal (B) or more rostral (C) levels, which yield reduced neural crest populations and tend to disaggregate or grow neurites. Abbreviations: n, neurites; nc, neural crest cells; nt, neural tube. Bar = 100 µm.

limited ability to migrate (*Figure 3B*) (see also ref. 7). Similarly, if neural tubes are obtained from more rostral regions where neural crest cells have almost achieved separation from the neural tube (region C in *Figure 2–1*), they produce very few neural crest cells, instead they grow numerous neurites out of the ventral region of the explant (*Figure 3C*).

3. The last condition to be met concerns the choice of an adequate substratum for explant anchorage and cellular motility. Although neural crest cells are able to emigrate from explants that have been deposited on plastic dishes designed for cell culture, the nature and composition of the substratum greatly influence both the number of emigrating cells, their viability, and the distance covered. Thus, fibronectin, vitronectin, and laminin promote extensive migration of neural crest cells (8–11). Conversely, polylysine, tenascin, and certain proteoglycans are poor substrata (12–14). Collagens can be used as substrata for neural crest cells, but only collagen types I and IV are efficient, the other types tested so far (types II, V, and VII) were found not to support motility. In addition, collagens are generally more efficient as native forms rather than denatured (9,15). In conclusion, the choice of a substratum for neural crest cells will depend largely on the final goal of the culture. If neural crest cells have to be produced in 'large' quantities, fibronectin, either purified and used at concentrations above 5 µg/ml or derived from serum, is certainly the simplest choice. Other substrata, e.g. laminin, will be more appropriate, however, if neuronal differentiation is needed.

Finally, it should be noted that other methods than that described in *Protocol 1* have been used to produce trunk neural crest cells (see, for example, ref. 16). They consist of dissecting out either the neural folds prior to neural crest cell emigration or the sclerotomes once they are invaded by neural crest cells. These methods are not commonly used and will not be described here in detail, essentially because they do not give rise to pure neural crest populations free of contaminants and also they require a great expertise in dissecting embryonic tissues.

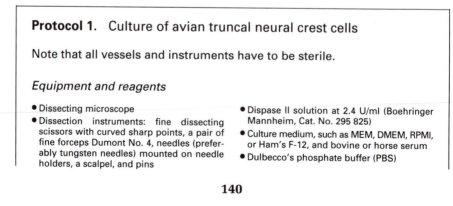

Protocol 1. Culture of avian truncal neural crest cells

Note that all vessels and instruments have to be sterile.

Equipment and reagents

- Dissecting microscope
- Dissection instruments: fine dissecting scissors with curved sharp points, a pair of fine forceps Dumont No. 4, needles (preferably tungsten needles) mounted on needle holders, a scalpel, and pins
- Dispase II solution at 2.4 U/ml (Boehringer Mannheim, Cat. No. 295 825)
- Culture medium, such as MEM, DMEM, RPMI, or Ham's F-12, and bovine or horse serum
- Dulbecco's phosphate buffer (PBS)

• Glass Petri dish containing a silicone elastomer (e.g. Rhodorsil from Rhône-Poulenc) which cross-links at room temperature to form an elastic material (follow the manufacturer's instructions for an appropriate preparation of the polymer), and into which animal charcoal is incorporated to make it opaque. The elastic properties of this material make it extremely convenient to pin embryos down for excision of tissue explants and its opacity allows to visualize the detailed structure of the animal. In addition, it can be sterilized and reused many times.

• Fibronectin, laminin, or vitronectin: these substratum molecules can be purchased from various suppliers (Gibco-BRL, Sigma, Collaborative Research, etc.) and should be used at concentrations ranging from 1–100 µg/ml in PBS (optimal coating concentrations are 10 µg/ml, 5 µg/ml, and 25 µg/ml for fibronectin, vitronectin, and laminin, respectively)

Method

1. Collecting the embryo. Incubate eggs for 2.5 days (60 h) at $37 \pm 1\,°C$ in an incubator. Cut the egg shell with curved dissecting scissors and transfer the yolk sterilely from the egg into PBS. Remove the embryo from the yolk by cutting the area opaca all around the embryo proper and collect it into PBS. Peel off the transparent vitelline membrane covering the embryo using a pair of fine forceps.

2. Dissecting the trunk portions (see *Figure 2–1*). Pin the embryo down in the elastomer-containing dish, determine the stage of development of the embryo (i.e. the total number of somite pairs), and with a scalpel dissect rectangular sections of tissues including the neural tube, the flanking somites, and lateral plates, as shown in *Figure 2–1*. Collect the explant in culture medium. In order to determine the number of somite pairs in embryos older than 25 somite pairs, it is not necessary to count all somites, but simply to count those situated caudally to the 21st somite where the large extraembryonic blood vessels are entering the embryo.

3. Dissecting the neural tube (see *Figure 2–2* to *2–4*). Incubate the trunk portions in dispase for about 30 min at room temperature. Dispase is a neutral protease that exhibits a number of advantages over other proteases such as trypsin, collagenase, and pronase:

   • it is stable and active at room temperature

   • it allows a gentle dissociation of tissues and does not damage cell membrane

   • it is inactivated simply by dilution

   • it is cheap

   After 30 min of incubation in dispase, tissues of the explants begin to separate, and dissection can start. First, peel off the ectoderm using a pair of needles. As shown in *Figure 2–2*, one of the needles (N1) maintains the bit of trunk in place while the other needle (N2) is introduced under the ectoderm and separates it from the neural tube. Then,

Protocol 1. *Continued*

remove the somites on either sides of the neural tubes as shown in *Figure 2–3*. Separate the neural tube from the endoderm. Finally, progressively dissociate the notochord from the neural tube as shown in *Figure 2–4*. Note that tissues are maintained in dispase during the whole process of dissection. When free of any contaminating tissues, neural tube explants are gently sucked in with a pipette and transferred into culture medium supplemented with 1% bovine serum. This allows the tissue to recover from the enzyme treatment. If serum-free cultures have to be made, however, serum can be omitted without any damage for the tissues.

4. After recovery, neural tubes are transferred into a culture dish previously coated with fibronectin, laminin, or vitronectin. Neural crest cells can be cultured in any kind of plastic dishes. However, we do not recommend 96-well culture dishes, because the wells are too deep and their edges are too steep for allowing an easy manipulation of the explant inside of the well. Conversely, 35 mm dishes and Terasaki plates are particularly appropriate. For coating, incubate the dish with the solution of substratum molecule at the desired dilution at 37 °C for 1 h, followed by several washes in PBS. For most molecules studied, adsorption to the plastic remains proportional to the coating concentration within the range of 0.1–50 µg/ml (10).

5. As neural tubes tend to float in the culture medium and may be displaced while transferring the dish into the incubator, we recommend allowing the neural tube to attach to the plastic before transferring to the incubator or, better, to place the explants into wells (e.g. of Terasaki plates) to avoid turbulence. In addition, small wells allow a rapid conditioning of the culture medium by the explants, thus favouring cell survival.

6. Neural tubes are usually cultured at 37 °C in a humidified 5% CO_2/95% air incubator in culture medium supplemented with 3–5% bovine or horse serum. They may also be cultured in serum-free medium containing 10 µg/ml insulin, 10 µg/ml transferrin, and 0.1% ovalbumin, or in more complex chemically defined media (see below).

2.1.2 Mammalian (mouse or rat)

While the avian model has permitted considerable advances in our understanding of neural crest cell migration and differentiation, the mouse embryo has attracted much interest recently because it offers many particular advantages. First, a variety of mutant strains have phenotypes that correspond to neurological defects linked with neural crest development. Secondly, the ability to obtain transgenic mice by introducing foreign or mutated genes into the germline allows the genetic manipulation of mouse embryogenesis. Finally, neural crest cells can be re-introduced into the embryo *in utero* where they participate in normal embryonic development (17).

Obtaining mouse or rat trunk neural crest cells is basically the same as for avian embryos (see *Protocol 1*) (18,19). Mouse and rat embryos are isolated at day 8.5–9 and day 10–10.5 of gestation, respectively (day of vaginal plug = day 0 of gestation), according to procedures described extensively in *Mammalian development: a practical approach* (ed. M. Monk) (see Chapter 3, by R. Beddington). After removal of placenta and fetal membranes using fine forceps, embryos are used for dissection of neural tubes essentially as described in *Protocol 1* for avian embryos. In particular, the choice of trunk regions to be excised and of the substratum molecules follow the same rules. Mammalian trunk neural crest cells can be incubated in DMEM or Ham's F-12 culture medium supplemented with 5–15% bovine serum or in serum-free chemically defined media (see below).

2.2 Chick cranial neural crest

In contrast to their trunk counterparts, cranial neural crest cells are abundant during migration at least in the avian embryo and are directly accessible for dissection. In addition, although it has been performed previously (see, for example, ref. 19), production of cranial neural crest cells using the same procedure as for trunk neural crest cells cannot be carried out easily, essentially because the neural tube has to be excised at stages when it is closing and, consequently, it does not keep its tubular shape, and only a limited number of neural crest cells are able to emigrate from it.

The principle of the procedure described in *Protocol 2* is to dissect out cranial neural crest cells together with its associated ectoderm and to put them directly in culture (*Figures 4* and *5*). Indeed, during migration, cranial neural crest cells form a sheet of several cell layers situated under the ectoderm and over the loose cranial mesenchyme. As it is dense and thick, this cell sheet is clearly visible in the intact embryo and can be excised as a whole (16,20). However, migration of neural crest cells in the cranial region is extremely rapid, therefore the timing at which they can be excised is very restricted. Accurate staging of embryos is thus critical to obtaining large amounts of neural crest cells. The embryos should be in the stage range of 8–12 somite pairs, 10 somites being best. Embryos older than 12 somite pairs should be discarded, because most neural crest cells have already reached the ventral regions of the animal, and there is a risk of excising mesodermal cells instead of neural crest cells. After dissection, cranial neural crest explants put in culture with the lining ectoderm readily adhere to the bottom of the culture dish and migration of cells from the periphery of the explant starts almost immediately. After 24 hours in culture, neural crest cells form an outgrowth of about 1000 to 2000 cells surrounding the ectoderm which

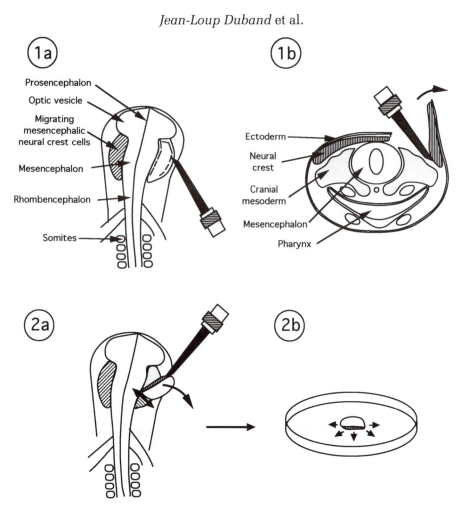

Figure 4. Dissection of cranial neural crest cells. (1) Schematic representation of the head region of a 10 somite embryo illustrating the migrating neural crest cells and the region to be dissected (dashed line). (a) Dorsal view and (b) transverse section showing how the needle has to be inserted under the explant to avoid collecting cranial mesoderm together with neural crest cells. (2) Diagram illustrating how the ectoderm and neural crest explant is peeled off (a) and put in culture in a dish (b).

retains its epithelial organization and can be removed from the dish with needles (*Figure 5B*). As the process of cranial neural crest cell appearance and migration is somewhat different in the mammalian embryo, essentially because of a different organization of the neural epithelium, the methodology for dissecting neural crest cells in *Protocol 2* cannot be applied to the mouse or rat.

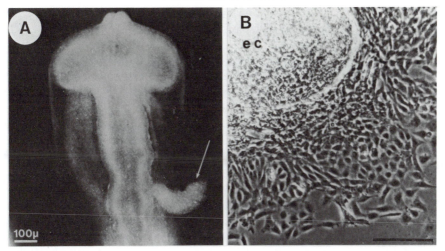

Figure 5. (A) Dorsal view of the cranial region of a 10 somite quail embryo showing a fragment of migrating neural crest that has been dissected out on the right side (*arrow*). (B) Morphology of cranial neural crest outgrowth after 24 hours in culture. Neural crest cells have migrated out of the initial explant and formed a dense colony of fibroblast-like cells at the periphery of the ectoderm (ec). Bar = 100 μm.

Protocol 2. Culture of avian cephalic neural crest cells

Equipment and reagents
- See *Protocol 1*

Method

1. Incubate eggs for about 36 h at 37 °C, and collect the embryos in PBS as described in *Protocol 1*. Peel off the vitelline membrane and determine the stage of development of the embryo with great care.

2. Excising neural crest cells (see *Figures 4* and *5A*). As shown in *Figure 4–1a* and in *Figure 5A*, with a sharp tungsten needle cut the ectoderm and underlying neural crest first laterally, then medially along the neural tube, and finally behind the optic vesicle. Take care not to go too deep into the embryo to avoid excising cranial mesodermal cells together with neural crest cells (*Figure 4–1b*). The last step, as illustrated in *Figure 4–2*, consists of peeling the ectoderm plus attached neural crest backwards with the needle and cut the last attached side.

3. After excision, the explant is immediately rinsed in PBS or in DMEM and placed in a tissue culture dish containing a small volume of culture medium. When, after several hours at 37 °C, the explants have attached to the bottom of the dish and have begun to flatten out, more culture medium is added. Alternatively, explants can be incubated in wells as described in *Protocol 1*.

---

3. Establishing conditions for differentiation of neural crest cells *in vitro*

The process of neural crest cell differentiation has been much studied *in vivo* in the avian embryo. This species is appropriate for this type of study because the embryo is accessible to experimentation in the egg during the entire period of development. Moreover, interspecific chimeras between quail and chick embryos and *in vivo* lineage tracing experiments using vital dyes, like DiI, have been instrumental in following the fate of neural crest cells throughout their developmental history and have demonstrated that individual neural crest cells are multipotent (1,21). Not only have these *in vivo* studies been useful for studying the normal development of neural crest derivatives, but also transplantations of tissues into ectopic sites have revealed that the embryonic microenvironment plays an essential role in the formation of the peripheral nervous system from the neural crest. However, *in vivo* studies only assess the fate of neural crest cells at a single time point and only address the question of progressive restriction of potentialities. They do not, however, allow a detailed analysis of the mechanism of action of differentiation factors. Therefore, different strategies have been developed to follow the fate of individual cells exposed to controlled environments *in vitro*. The recent demonstration of the existence of multipotent neural crest stem cells is certainly the most spectacular result obtained with such *in vitro* approaches (22).

3.1 Cloning neural crest cells

Since the pioneering work of Cohen and Konigsberg (4), several successful attempts have been made to clone avian or mammalian neural crest cells (22–24).

3.1.1 Basic cloning technique

Protocol 3. Cloning of neural crest cells

Equipment and reagents
- See *Protocol 1*

Method

1. Cultures of cranial or truncal neural crest cells are generated from quail or mouse embryos as described in *Protocols 1* and *2*.

2. After 18–24 h in culture, neural tubes or ectoderms are carefully removed from the dishes with tungsten needles and discarded. Remaining, attached neural crest cells are dissociated into a single cell suspension after a 3–5-min treatment at 37 °C with a solution of

---

146

0.025% trypsin, 0.02% EDTA in PBS and, after addition of an equal volume of culture medium supplemented with 5% bovine serum, they are centrifuged for 5 min at 1000 r.p.m. (150g).

3. Cells are resuspended in fresh culture medium, counted, and plated into dishes so that the density of the cell population does not exceed 200–250 cells/100 mm diameter dish.

4. Cells are allowed to attach to the dish and individual cells are identified with an inverted microscope equipped with a x 4 objective lens, and marked by inscribing a circle around them with a pencil on the underside of the dish.

5. After identification, cells are fed every other day for two to three weeks. Typically, clones of several hundred cells to several thousands of cells are obtained after 10–15 days in culture.

6. Subcloning of the colonies. Clones of interest are examined microscopically to ensure that there are no impinging colonies. Sterile glass cloning cylinders with an inner diameter not exceeding 3 mm (Corning) are coated on one end with silicone grease and placed around the clone, and cells are collected from the cylinder after trypsin treatment as described at step 2. Cells are centrifuged for 5 min at 1000 r.p.m. (150g), resuspended in fresh medium, and are plated again in dishes.

3.1.2 A valuable variant cloning technique

As the cloning procedure described in *Protocol 3* may not allow the full differentiation potential of neural crest cells, because a significant proportion of the clones does not develop, another approach has been proposed to allow both a faster cycling and a greater survival of the cloned cells (24). The methodology is essentially the same as the one described in *Protocol 3* with the following two modifications. First, colonies are not obtained by the limited dilution method but result from individual cells that are taken from a single cell suspension with a micropipette under microscopic control using a x 10 objective lens. Secondly, instead of being plated on 100 mm plastic dishes, single neural crest cells are deposited on established feeder layers of mouse Swiss 3T3 fibroblasts cultured in 4-well plates whose growth has been arrested by treatment for 2–3 h with mitomycin at 4 µg/ml (Sigma). Under these conditions, neural crest cells grow significantly faster than on plastic and the clonal efficiency is considerably higher. In addition, cells can be easily distinguished morphologically from the 3T3 cells.

3.2 Factors affecting neural crest cell differentiation

3.2.1 Chemically defined media

Since the original studies of Le Douarin and coworkers (16,20), it has become clear that both the composition of the culture medium and the nature of the substratum are critical for obtaining almost the full-range of neural crest derivatives *in vitro*. In particular, it was found that neuronal differentiation occurs at significantly higher levels in serum-deprived medium and that the phenotype exhibited by neural crest cells is under the influence of growth factors present in the culture medium. Therefore, several investigators have adapted prototypic chemically defined media for obtaining the largest possible range of derivatives from avian or mammalian neural crest cells (20,22,25). The compositions of two of them are given below.

(a) Ham's F-12 nutrient mixture supplemented with 2 mg/ml bovine serum albumin, 2.38 mg/ml Hepes, 50 μg/ml gentamycin, 0.1 μg/ml cortisol, 1 ng/ml insulin, 0.4 ng/ml 3,3′,5-triiodothyronine, 0.2 ng/ml parathyroid hormone, 0.01 ng/ml glucagon, 10 μg/ml transferrin, 0.1 ng/ml epidermal growth factor (EGF), and 0.2 ng/ml fibroblast growth factor (FGF).

(b) Leibovitz L-15 nutrient mixture supplemented with 1 mg/ml bovine serum albumin, 16 μg/ml putrescine, 6.3 μg/ml progesterone, 30 nM selenic acid, 39 pg/ml dexamethasone, 35 ng/ml retinoic acid, 5 μg/ml α-d, 1-tocopherol, 63 μg/ml β-hydroxybutyrate, 25 ng/ml cobalt chloride, 1 μg/ml biotin, 10 ng/ml oleic acid, 3.6 mg/ml glycerol, 100 ng/ml α-melanocyte-stimulating hormone, 10 ng/ml prostaglandin E1, 5 μg/ml insulin, 67.5 ng/ml 3,3′,5-triiodothyronine, 100 μg/ml transferrin, 100 ng/ml EGF, 4 ng/ml FGF, and 20 ng/ml 2.5S nerve growth factor (NGF).

All chemicals can be purchased from Sigma, Gibco-BRL, Calbiochem, or Boehringer Mannheim. We recommend they be prepared as 100 × stock solutions and stored at –80 °C. Chemically defined media are generally supplemented with 2–10% chick embryo extract to favour more complete differentiation of neural crest cells into their major derivatives, either in mass culture or under clonal conditions. Thus, sensory neurons, glial and Schwann cells, sympathetic neurons, adrenal chromaffin cells, and melanocytes can be obtained from avian or mammalian trunk neural crest cells, while the same derivatives in addition to cholinergic neurons and cartilage are generated by cranial neural crest cells (see, for example, refs 22 and 26).

Protocol 4.   Preparation of chick embryo extract

1. Chicken eggs are incubated for 11 days at 37 °C. Note that 'chick' embryo extract can also be prepared from nine-day quail embryos! Embryos are removed from the egg as described in *Protocol 1* and placed into a 100 mm Petri dish containing approx. 10 ml of culture medium at 4 °C.

2. Mince the embryos in the culture medium with a pair of fine scissors. Collect the culture medium and the minced embryos in a 20 ml syringe and homogenize the whole mixture by thorough passages

through the syringe. Add more culture medium if the solution becomes too viscous.

3. Once an homogeneous mixture is obtained, add more culture medium to a final volume of 50 ml. Approximately ten embryos are sufficient to prepare 50 ml of chick embryo extract. Centrifuge the mixture at 30 000 *g* for 5 h at 4 °C. Discard the pellet, collect the supernatant, pass it though a 0.45 μm filter, and store it at −80 °C until use.

3.2.2 Growth factors

Table 3 gives a list of the major growth factors that have been shown either to promote the survival and division of 'immature' neural crest cells or to induce their differentiation into a given lineage. The roles of these factors have been analysed, in most cases, in mass cultures of neural crest cells and, in fewer cases, under clonal conditions (reviewed in ref. 27). It should be emphasized that growth factors known to exert a trophic activity only on *fully differentiated* cells deriving from the neural crest are not listed in this table. Only those affecting survival, division, and differentiation of neural crest cells and of committed progenitors are considered.

3.3 Markers of neural crest cell differentiation

The analysis of neural crest cell differentiation has been made possible in recent years because a battery of markers for each lineage has been developed. *Table 4* gives a list of such markers. This list is not exhaustive, but will

Table 3. Growth factors affecting neural crest cell division, survival, and differentiation[a]

Factor[a]	Concentration	Effect[b]	Reference
bFGF	0.01–1 ng/ml	S on early NCC	28
	0.1–1 ng/ml	D of early NCC into neurons	29
	10 ng/ml	D of SA progenitors into sympathetic neurons	30
EGF	0.01–10 μg/ml	M on early NCC	31
BDNF	10 ng/ml	D of early NCC into sensory neurons	23
LIF	100 U/ml	D of early NCC into sensory neurons	32
NT3	0.1–10 ng/ml	M on early NCC	33
	10 ng/ml	D of sensory progenitors into neurons	34
IGF-1	1–100 ng/ml	D of early NCC into SA progenitors	35
α-MSH	0.1 μg/ml	D of early NCC into melanocytes	36
SLF	100 ng/ml	M on melanocyte progenitors	37
GGF	0.1–10 nM	D of early NCC into glia	38

[a] Abbreviations: bFGF, basic fibroblast growth factor; EGF, epidermal growth factor; BDNF, brain-derived neurotrophic factor; LIF, leukaemia inhibitory factor; NT3, neurotrophin 3; IGF-1, insulin-like growth factor-1; α-MSH, α-melanocyte-stimulating hormone; SLF, steel factor; GGF, glial growth factor.
[b] Abbreviations: M, mitogenic-promoting activity; S, survival-promoting activity; D, differentiation-promoting activity; early NCC, undifferentiated neural crest cells; SA, sympathoadrenal.

Table 4. Markers for neural crest cells and their derivatives

Marker[a]	Molecular nature	Cell type specificity	Species specificity	Antibody[b]
NC-1/HNK-1	Carbohydrate moiety	Neural crest cells and all neural derivatives	Birds, certain mammals	Caltag/Immunotech
NF 160	Intermediate filament	All neurons	Birds, mammals	Immunotech
A2B5	Glycolipid	All neurons	Birds	Ref. 39
SSEA-1	Carbohydrate moiety	All sensory neurons	Birds	Ref. 40
		Some sensory neurons	Rat	
Subst. P	Neuropeptide	Sensory neurons	Birds	Chemicon
		Sensory, autonomic neurons	Mammals	
VIP	Neuropeptide	Sympathetic, sensory neurons	Birds, mammals	Chemicon
CGRP	Neuropeptide	Sensory neurons	Birds, mammals	Chemicon
SN1	Unknown	Some sensory neurons	Birds	Ref. 41
TH	Enzyme	Adrenergic neurons	Birds, mammals	Chemicon
DBH	Enzyme	Adrenergic neurons	Birds, mammals	Chemicon
ChAT	Enzyme	Cholinergic neurons	Birds, mammals	Chemicon
GFAP	Intermediate filament	Glial cells	Birds, mammals	Sigma
SMP	Surface glycoprotein	Schwann cells	Birds	Ref. 42
MEBL-1	Surface glycoprotein	Melanocytes	Birds	Ref. 43
Mash1[c]	Transcription factor	Sympathetic neurons	Mouse	Ref. 44
c-ret[c] receptor	Tyrosine kinase	Enteric, sympathetic neurons	Mouse	Ref. 45

[a] Abbreviations: HNK-1, human natural killer-1; NF 160, neurofilament 160K; SSEA-1, stage-specific embryonic antigen 1; Subst. P, substance P; VIP, vasointestinal peptide; CGRP, calcitonin gene-related peptide; TH, tyrosine hydroxylase; DBH, dopamine-β-hydroxylase; ChAT, choline acetyltransferase; GFAP, gliary fibrillary acidic protein; SMP, Schwann cell myelin protein.
[b] When the antibody is, to our knowledge, not commercially available, a reference is given for greater details on the characterization of the antibody.
[c] *Mash1* and *c-ret* are two genes that encode a transcription factor and a tyrosine kinase receptor, respectively, and that have been detected by *in situ* hybridization in a number of neural crest derivatives and that can be appropriately used to follow neural crest cell differentiation into sympathetic and enteric ganglia.

facilitate neural crest cell differentiation to be followed *in vitro*. Two genes, *Mash1* and *c-ret*, have been included within the list to take into account the recent progress made in the discovery of genes that are specifically expressed in neural crest lineages.

Acknowledgements

We are extremely grateful to Mireille Fauquet for providing micrographs. Work of the authors is supported by the Centre National de la Recherche Scientifique (Programme ATIPE), the Ministère de la Recherche et de la Technologie (91.T.0011), the Association pour la Recherche contre le Cancer (ARC-6517), the Institut National de la Santé et de la Recherche Médicale (CRE 910705), the Association Française contre les Myopathies, and the Fondation pour la Recherche Médicale. M. D. and F. M. are recipients of a predoctoral fellowship of the Ministère de l'Enseignement Supérieur et de la Recherche.

References

1. Le Douarin, N. M. (1982). *The neural crest*. Cambridge University Press, Cambridge.
2. Le Douarin, N. M., Ziller, C., and Couly, G. F. (1993). *Dev. Biol.*, **159,** 24.
3. Anderson, D. J. (1989). *Neuron*, **3,** 1.
4. Cohen, A. M. and Konigsberg, I. R. (1975). *Dev. Biol.*, **46,** 262.
5. Vincent, M. and Thiery, J. P. (1984). *Dev. Biol.*, **103,** 468.
6. Newgreen, D. F., Powell, M. E., and Moser, B. (1990). *Dev. Biol.*, **139,** 100.
7. Delannet, M. and Duband, J.-L. (1992). *Development*, **116,** 275.
8. Rovasio, R. A., Delouvée, A., Yamada, K. M., Timpl, R., and Thiery, J. P. (1983). *J. Cell Biol.*, **96,** 462.
9. Tucker, R. P. and Erickson, C. A. (1984). *Dev. Biol.*, **104,** 390.
10. Perris, R., Paulsson, M., and Bronner-Fraser, M. (1989). *Dev. Biol.*, **136,** 222.
11. Delannet, M., Martin, F., Bossy, B., Cheresh, D. A., Reichardt, L. F., and Duband, J.-L. (1994). *Development*, **120,** 2687.
12. Mackie, E. J., Tucker, R. P., Halfter, W., Chiquet-Ehrismann, R., and Epperlein, H. H. (1988). *Development*, **102,** 237.
13. Tan, S. S., Crossin, K. L., Hoffman, S., and Edelman, G. M. (1987). *Proc. Natl. Acad. Sci. USA*, **84,** 7977.
14. Perris, R. and Johansson, S. (1990). *Dev. Biol.*, **137,** 1.
15. Perris, R., Krotoski, D., and Bronner-Fraser, M. (1991). *Development*, **113,** 969.
16. Fauquet, M., Smith, J., Ziller, C., and Le Douarin, N. M. (1981). *J. Neurosci.*, **1,** 478.
17. Jaenisch, R. (1985). *Nature*, **318,** 181.
18. Boisseau, S. and Simonneau, M. (1989). *Development*, **106,** 665.
19. Newgreen, D. F. and Thiery, J. P. (1980). *Cell Tiss. Res.*, **211,** 269.
20. Ziller, C., Dupin, E., Brazeau, P., Paulin, D., and Le Douarin, N. M. (1983). *Cell*, **32,** 627.

21. Bronner-Fraser, M. and Fraser, S. (1989). *Neuron*, **3,** 755.
22. Stemple, D. L. and Anderson, D. J. (1992). *Cell*, **71,** 973.
23. Sieber-Blum, M. (1991). *Neuron*, **6,** 949.
24. Baroffio, A., Dupin, E., and Le Douarin, N. M. (1988). *Proc. Natl. Acad. Sci. USA*, **85,** 5325.
25. Sieber-Blum, M. and Chokshi, H. R. (1985). *Exp. Cell Res.*, **158,** 267.
26. Baroffio, A., Dupin, E., and Le Douarin, N. M. (1991). *Development*, **112,** 301.
27. Stemple, D. L. and Anderson, D. J. (1993). *Dev. Biol.*, **159,** 12.
28. Kalcheim, C. (1989). *Dev. Biol.*, **134,** 1.
29. Brill, G., Vaisman, N., Neufeld, G., and Kalcheim, C. (1992). *Development*, **115,** 1059.
30. Birren, S. J. and Anderson, D. J. (1990). *Neuron*, **4,** 189.
31. Erickson, C. A. and Turley, E. A. (1987). *Exp. Cell Res.*, **169,** 267.
32. Murphy, M., Reid, K., Hilton, D. J., and Bartlett, P. F. (1991). *Proc. Natl. Acad. Sci. USA*, **88,** 3498.
33. Kalcheim, C., Carmeli, C., and Rosenthal, A. (1992). *Proc. Natl. Acad. Sci. USA*, **89,** 1661.
34. Wright, E. M., Vogel, K. S., and Davies, A. M. (1992). *Neuron*, **9,** 1.
35. Xue, Z.-G., Le Douarin, N. M., and Smith, J. (1988). *Cell Differ. Dev.*, **25,** 1.
36. Satoh, M. and Ide, H. (1987). *Dev. Biol.*, **119,** 579.
37. Murphy, M., Reid, K., Williams, D. E., Lyman, S. D., and Bartlett, P. F. (1992). *Dev. Biol.*, **153,** 396.
38. Shah, N. M., Marchionni, M. A., Isaacs, I., Stroobant, P., and Anderson, D. J. (1994). *Cell*, **77,** 349.
39. Vogel, K. S. and Weston, J. A. (1988). *Neuron*, **1,** 569.
40. Sieber-Blum, M. (1989). *Dev. Biol.*, **134,** 362.
41. Marusich, M. F., Pourmehr, K., and Weston, J. A. (1986). *Dev. Biol.*, **118,** 494.
42. Dulac, C., Cameron-Curry, P., Ziller, C., and Le Douarin, N. M. (1988). *Neuron*, **1,** 211.
43. Kitamura, K., Takiguchi-Hayashi, K., Sezaki, M., Yamamoto, H., and Takeuchi, T. (1992). *Development*, **114,** 367.
44. Guillemot, F., Lo, L.-C., Johnson, J. E., Auerbach, A. B., Anderson, D. J., and Joyner, A. L. (1993). *Cell*, **75,** 463.
45. Pachnis, V., Mankoo, B., and Costantini, F. (1993). *Development*, **119,** 1005.

12

Cranial sensory neurons

ALUN M. DAVIES

1. Introduction

Cranial sensory neurons have many advantages for studying the different phases of neuronal development. These neurons and their progenitor cell populations are well defined and can be easily obtained for *in vitro* experimental studies and are accessible to experimental manipulation *in ovo* in avian embryos from the earliest stages of their development (1,2). The peripheral target fields of several cranial sensory ganglia, such as the trigeminal ganglion, are clearly circumscribed, and this has facilitated detailed studies of the influence of the target field on various aspects of neuronal development (3–6). In contrast to the functional heterogeneity of dorsal root ganglia, cranial sensory neurons are for the most part segregated into functionally distinct populations. Perhaps as a consequence of this functional segregation, populations of cranial sensory neurons have quite distinct neurotrophic factor requirements. This has facilitated studies of the function and co-operation of different neurotrophic factors in regulating neuronal survival (7–9).

In this chapter I shall describe techniques for culturing the different populations of embryonic chicken cranial sensory neurons and selected populations of embryonic mouse cranial sensory neurons. I shall restrict my description to the establishment of dissociated cultures because, unlike explant cultures, the effects of various factors on neuronal survival are easily quantified in low density cultures. Also, because non-neuronal cells can be effectively removed from these cultures, the analysis of the effects of a particular factor on neurons is not complicated by any indirect effects mediated by non-neuronal cells.

2. Dissection techniques

All dissections and subsequent preparation of neuronal cultures should be carried out in a laminar flow hood using standard sterile technique. For the final stages of dissection, a good quality stereomicroscope with zoom lens is essential. A fibre-optic light source should be used for illumination as this

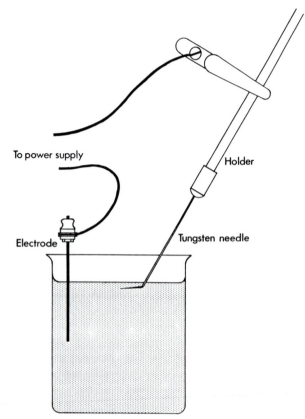

Figure 1. Method for making tungsten needles. Modified from ref. 22.

avoids overheating the specimen. Tungsten needles are required to complete dissections and to remove adherent connective tissue from the dissected neural tissue. These are made from 0.5 mm diameter tungsten wire as follows (*Figure 1*).

Protocol 1. Making tungsten needles

Equipment and reagents

- Toothed forceps, straight and curved watchmaker's forceps, scalpels—forceps and scalpels should be sterilized by either autoclaving, dry heat, or flaming in alcohol
- Sterile plastic Petri dishes (60 and 100 mm diameter)

- All dissections are best carried out in L-15 medium without sodium bicarbonate—it is not necessary to add a buffer like Hepes to this medium

Method

1. Cut the wire into 3–5 cm lengths using a grind wheel.

2. Bend the end 1 cm by an angle of about 60°.

---

3. Immerse this end with the bent portion near horizontal in 1 M KOH.

4. Pass a 3–12 V AC current through the wire and a second electrode (copper or steel rod) immersed in this solution. The tungsten is etched away over several minutes forming a taper from the bend to the tip of the needle.

5. To form a sharp point at the tip, place the bent portion vertically in the solution for several seconds.

6. Wash the needles in water to remove the alkali.

7. For dissection, the needles are conveniently held in chuck-grip platinum wire holders. Sterilize tungsten needles in a Bunsen burner flame.

2.1 Early cranial sensory ganglia from chicken embryos

Because the peripheral and central axons of different cranial sensory ganglia have markedly different distances to grow to reach their targets during development, cultures of cranial sensory neurons at the stage when their axons would normally be growing to their targets *in vivo* have been very useful for studying differences in *de novo* axonal growth rate and the onset of neurotrophic factor dependence in relation to differences in the timing of target field innervation (1,2). The trigeminal, geniculate, vestibular, petrosal, and nodose ganglia, which contain neurons derived from neurogenic placodes, can be dissected from chicken embryos as early as E3 (Hamburger-Hamilton stages 19–21) (10). This is carried out as in *Protocol 2*.

Protocol 2. Dissection of early cranial sensory ganglia

1. Incubate fertile chicken eggs in a forced-draft, humidifed incubator at 38 °C for the required time. To remove embryos from eggs, hold the egg with blunt end uppermost (where the airspace is located). Swab this with 70% alcohol and allow it to dry. Crack the shell in a line around the airspace by tapping with forceps and remove this portion of the shell and the membrane lining the airspace. Carefully remove the embryo together with its adherent membranes with a pair of curved forceps.

2. Wash the embryos in a Petri dish containing L-15 medium and remove all membranes with pairs of watchmaker's forceps. Transfer the embryos to a 60 mm Petri dish containing L-15 medium. Small embryos can be best transferred without damage by carefully aspirating them into the blunt end of a Pasteur pipette. To facilitate visualization of early ganglia within the partially dissected embryonic head (below), carry out the dissection on a black background with

Protocol 2. *Continued*

illumination from above. Placing a small volume of liquid between the Petri dish and the underlying black background will improve the contrast.

3. Use tungsten needles to make two transverse cuts to isolate the part of the developing head that contains the trigeminal, geniculate, vestibular, petrosal, and nodose ganglia (*Figure 2*).

4. Bisect this part of the head along the saggital plane. Do this by inserting a tungsten needle into the cavity of the developing fourth ventricle and orientate the tissue so that its dorsal aspect lies next to the bottom of the Petri dish. Then press against the bottom of the culture dish with the inserted tungsten needle to cut through the roof of the fourth ventricle. Then orient the tissue so that its ventral aspect now faces the bottom of the Petri dish. Complete the bisection by pushing a tungsten down through the tissue to the bottom of the dish.

5. Use a tungsten needle to remove the hindbrain from the medial aspect of each half of the bisected tissue. With the tissue lying on its side, it will be possible to make out the ganglia (which are slightly more opaque than the surrounding tissues) in the positions illustrated in *Figure 2*. The novice may find this difficult at E3. For this reason, I would recommend some practice using E4 embryos in which the ganglia can be seen more clearly.

6. Dissect the ganglia from the surrounding tissues by bringing two tungsten needles down on either side of each ganglion and remove any adherent connective tissue with these needles.

7. Collect each kind of ganglion in a separate 35 mm Petri dish. Transfer the ganglia to these dishes using a siliconized Pasteur pipette. The tendency of the ganglia to stick to the inside of the pipette can be discouraged by first rinsing the pipette with some serum-containing medium. Place the collection Petri dishes on a dark background so that you can confirm that the ganglia have left the pipette tip.

2.2 Mid-embryonic cranial sensory neurons from chicken embryos

Naturally occurring cell death occurs in cranial sensory ganglia during the mid-embryonic stages. Because each population of cranial sensory neurons is dependent on a particular neurotrophic factor or combination of factors, studying these neurons at this stage of development has been useful for analysing the function and co-operation of neurotrophic factors (7,9,11,12). The location of the cranial sensory ganglia in the E10 chick embryo is shown in *Figure 3*.

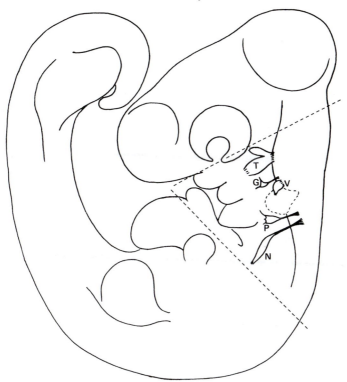

Figure 2. Lateral aspect of a stage 21 (E3.5) chicken embryo showing the location of the two transverse incisions (interrupted lines) used to isolate the region of the developing head that contains the trigeminal (T), geniculate (G), vestibulo-acoustic (V), petrosal (P), and nodose ganglia (N). The central nerve branches of the ganglia are shown in all cases.

2.2.1 Nodose ganglia

The ganglia are located either side of the midline in tissues lying in front of the vertebral column at the base of the neck.

Protocol 3. Isolation of nodose ganglia

1. Extract embryos from eggs using a pair of curved forceps placed beneath the neck and decapitate the embryos close the the base of the skull.

2. Remove the skin from the front of the neck and upper thorax using a pair of watchmaker's forceps, and expose the great vessels emerging from the heart by separating the overlying muscular and skeletal tissues at the upper part of the thorax.

3. Insert one blade of a watchmaker's forceps deep to the root of the

---

Protocol 3. *Continued*

great vessel (i.e. between these and the underlying vertebral column). Grasp the great vessels and sever their attachment to the heart using a second pair of watchmaker's forceps. Gently pull the great vessels and the attached tissues lying in front of the neck away from the underlying vertebral column, using the second pair of forceps to loosen the tissues so that they peal away from the vertebral column without tearing (*Figure 4*).

4. Harvest this tissue, which contains both nodose ganglia, in a fresh 65 mm Petri dish containing L-15 medium. Subdissect this tissue using tungsten needles. The nodose ganglia are easily recognized by their glistening white appearance, spindle shape, and attached vagus nerve. Remove the vagus nerves and clean the ganglia of any adherent tissue.

2.2.2 Other cranial sensory ganglia

The other cranial sensory ganglia are dissected from the cranial base after removal of the brain.

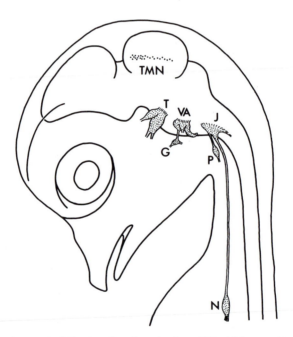

Figure 3. Lateral aspect of the head and neck of an E10 chicken embryo showing the locations of the trigeminal mesencephalic nucleus (TMN) and the trigeminal (T), geniculate (G), vestibulo-acoustic (V), petrosal (P), jugular (J), and nodose ganglia (N). Modified from ref. 11.

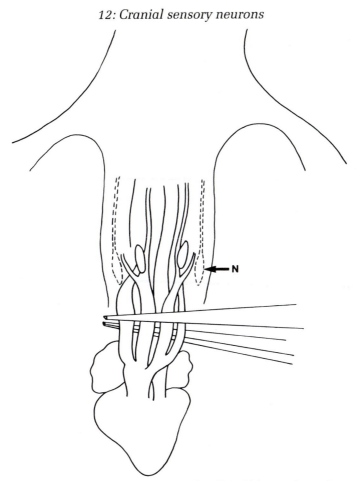

Figure 4. Ventral aspect of the thoracic region of an E10 chicken embryo after removal of the skin and reflection of the ventral thoracic wall to either side of the midline, exposing the heart and great vessels. The great vessels are clasped with a pair of forceps prior to removing the attached tissues lying above and in front of the upper thorax and lower neck. The connective tissue lying either side of the great vessels contains the two nodose ganglia (N) attached to the vagus nerves (shown by the interrupted lines).

Protocol 4. Dissection of other cranial sensory glia

1. After decapitation, remove the cranial vault with watchmaker's forceps, taking care not to damage the underlying brain if this is required for dissection of the trigeminal mesencephalic nucleus (see below).

2. Carefully remove the brain by passing a small spatula between it and the base of the skull.

3. Use a number 15 scapel blade to bisect the cranial base in the sagittal

Protocol 4. *Continued*

plane and subdissect the resulting half bases along the lines shown in *Figure 5*.

4. Use tungsten needles to dissect the various ganglia from these tissue blocks. In each case the ganglia are easily identified by their characteristic shape (*Figure 3*). Take particular care to distinguish the spindle-shaped petrosal ganglion from the larger, medially situated superior cervical ganglion which has a rhomboidal shape.

5. Use tungsten needles to subdissect the trigeminal ganglion into regions containing the neural crest-derived, NGF-dependent, dorsomedial neurons and the placode-derived, BDNF-dependent ventrolateral neurons (*Figure 6*). Between 20 and 30 ganglia are required in a standard preparation.

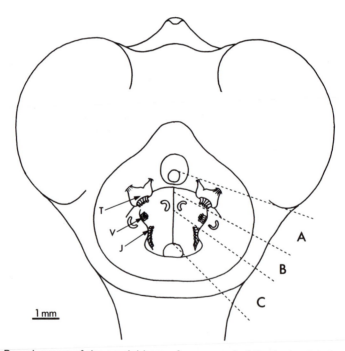

Figure 5. Dorsal aspect of the cranial base after removal of the brain showing the lines for subdissecting this tissue into blocks that contain the trigeminal ganglion (block A), vestibulo-acoustic and geniculate ganglia (block B), and the jugular and petrosal ganglia (block C). The trigeminal ganglion (T) and the roots of the vestibulo-acoustic (V) and jugular (J) ganglia are shown. Modified from ref. 22.

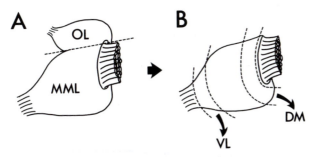

Figure 6. Subdissection of the trigeminal ganglion into dorsomedial (DM) and ventrolateral (VL) poles. The ophthalmic lobe (OL) is separated from the maxillo-mandibular lobe (MML) along the interrupted line shown in (A). The MML is subdissected along the lines shown in (B) to obtain the DM and VL poles. From ref. 22.

2.2.3 Trigeminal mesencephalic nucleus (TMN)

This population of neural crest-derived, BDNF-dependent, primary sensory neurons is dissected from the midbrain (13).

Protocol 5. Dissection of TMN

1. Collect brains in L-15 medium (20 to 40 in a standard preparation).
2. Transfer these to a fresh plastic Petri dish containing L-15 and complete the dissection with tungsten needles as shown in *Figure 7*.
3. Isolate the midbrain by two coronal incisions.
4. Carefully peel the pia mater off the midbrain starting on the ventral aspect. Take particular care to avoid tearing the roof of the cerebral aqueduct in which the TMN lies.
5. Dissect the roof the cerebral aqueduct from the midbrain and subdissect the median part of the TMN (in which the neurons are most densely packed) from this.

2.3 Trigeminal ganglia from mouse embryos

As with cranial sensory neurons in chicken embryos, the dissection technique for mouse embryo trigeminal ganglia differs with embryonic age. In all cases, however, the embryos have to be removed from pregnant females under sterile conditions.

Protocol 6. Isolation of mouse embryos

1. Kill the pregnant female at the required stage of gestation by cervical dislocation.
2. Squirt 70% alcohol from a wash bottle on the abdomen.

Protocol 6. *Continued*

3. Make a small incision in the skin on the front of the abdomen and grasp the skin just above and below the incision between the index finger and thumb of each hand. Pull the skin away from the incision, thereby tearing it and exposing the underlying abominal muscles.

4. Hold the the anterior abdominal muscle with a pair of toothed forceps and make a small incision with a pair of fine scissors, taking care not to cut into the intestines. Once air has entered the peritoneal cavity through this hole, the incision can be easily extended without fear of cutting the intestines and contaminating the dissection with bacteria.

5. Remove each gravid uterine horn by holding with a pair of toothed forceps and cutting it free with a pair of scissors.

6. To remove E9 to E12 embryos from the uterine horns, use a pair of fine-toothed forceps to pinch a small part of the musculature on the anti-mesometrial border of the uterine horn next to each embryo and snip this off with a pair of fine scissors. With practice, a hole of suffi- cient size can be made through which the embryo contained within intact chorion and amnion will be extruded by contraction of the remaining uterine muscle. Removing early embryos from the uterus within their membranes minimizes damage that would otherwise occur if naked embryos are forcibly extruded by muscular contraction through a hole in the uterine wall. Removal of E13 and older embryos within their membranes from the uterine horns is much more straightforward. To do this, make one continuous incision along the anti-mesometrial border of each uterine horn to expose the embryos enclosed within their membranes.

7. Detach the embryos still within their membranes from the uterine horns by plucking them off with a pair of watchmaker's forceps. Transfer these to a fresh 65 mm Petri dish containing L-15 medium and remove the chorion and amnion using watchmaker's forceps.

8. Transfer the embryos to a fresh 65 mm Petri dish containing L-15 medium. For very young embryos this is best done by aspirating the embryos into the blunt end of a Pasteur pipette (after the elongated, narrow part of the pipette has been carefully broken off so that the end of the wide part of the pipette can be inserted into a pipette bulb).

Protocol 7. Dissection of trigeminal ganglia from E10 to E12 embryos

1. Using tungsten needles, make two coronal incisions through the head, one just above the eye, the other between the maxillary and mandibular processes of the first branchial arch (*Figure 8a*). The

trigeminal ganglia can be seen as two opaque structures in the tissue slice obtained (*Figure 8b*).

2. The ganglia can be easily removed from the tissue slice and freed of any adherent mesenchymal tissue using tungsten needles. To free the ganglion of this tissue, use one needle to steady the ganglion and use the other to pinch off the adherent tissue against the bottom of the Petri dish.

3. Use a Pasteur pipette to transfer dissected ganglia to a 35 mm Petri dish containing L-15 medium until the required number has been obtained.

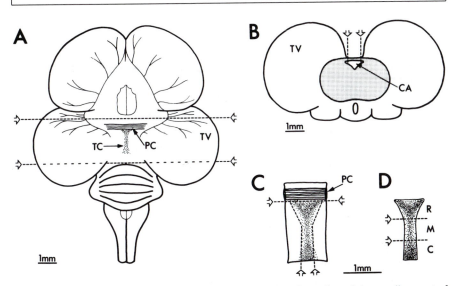

Figure 7. Drawings showing the successive stages in the dissection of the median part of the TMN from an E12 chicken embryo brain. (A) Dorsal aspect of the brain showing the location of the two coronal incisions (interrupted lines) for isolating the midbrain. (B) Caudal aspect of the isolated midbrain showing the location of the two parasagittal incisions for removing the roof of the cerebral aqueduct after carefully stripping off the overlying pia mater. (C) Dorsal aspect of the roof of the cerebral aqueduct showing the location of the incisions for cutting out the median part of the TMN. Tectal vesicle (TV), tectal commissure (TC), posterior commissure (PC), cerebral aqueduct (CA). From ref. 13.

Dissection of trigeminal ganglia from E13 and older embryos is similar to that of earlier ganglia except that a pair of fine scissors is used in the early stages of the dissection to cut through the cartilage (or bone in late fetal stages) of the developing head. The best pair of scissors for this dissection has very fine serrations along the blades which help grip the tissue to stop it from sliding out of the blades.

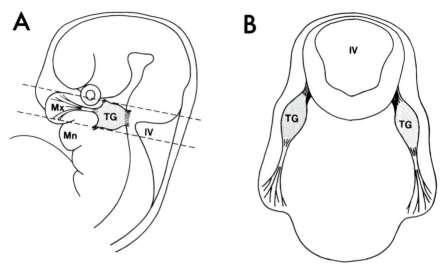

Figure 8. Drawings showing the dissection of the trigeminal ganglia from an E11 mouse embryo. (A) Lateral aspect of the E11 head showing the location of the transverse incisions (interrupted lines) for obtaining a slice of tissue that contains both trigeminal ganglia. (B) Rostral aspect of this slice showing the location of the trigeminal ganglia. Trigeminal ganglion (TG), maxillary process (Mx), mandibular process (Mn), fourth ventricle (IV). Modified from ref. 23.

Protocol 8.   Dissection of trigeminal ganglia from E13 and older embryos

1. Using a pair of forceps to steady the embryo, cut off the top of the skull in a plane just above the eyes and whisker pads.
2. Make a second cut parallel to the first passing through the mouth.
3. Transfer the tissue slices to a fresh 65 mm Petri dish containing L-15 medium and make two further cuts with the pair of scissors in front and behind the trigeminal ganglia (which are in a similar position to those illustrated in *Figure 8b*).
4. Transfer these pieces of tissues to a fresh 65 mm Petri dish containing L-15 medium and use tungsten needles to free the ganglia from the surrounding tissues and remove any adherent connective tissue.

2.4 Nodose ganglia from mouse embryos

In contrast to avian embryos, the nodose ganglion (otherwise known as the inferior vagal ganglion) remains situated close to the base of the skull. The dissection is similar at all ages except that a pair of fine scissors is required of the initial stages of the dissection in E13 and older embryos.

Protocol 9. Dissection of nodode ganglia

1. Remove the top of the skull and underlying forebrain using the same plane of section described for the first incision of the trigeminal dissection.

2. Decapitate the embryo and cut the head in half along the saggital plane (use tungsten needles up to E12 and a pair of scissors or a number 15 scalpel in E13 and older embyros).

3. Use tungsten needles to remove the hindbrain from the bisected head.

4. Open up the slit-like jugular foramen to the midline (*Figure 9*). For E12 and E13 embryos do this by inserting one tungsten needle into the jugular foramen so that it lies beneath the base of the skull lying medial to the foramen and bring a second needle into apposition with the first so as to cut through the intervening tissues. For older embryos use a pair of iridectomy scissors to accomplish this.

5. Use a pair of tungsten needles to open up the 'mouths' of the jugular foramen which will reveal the nodose ganglion lying in the base of this foramen. The nodose ganglion is an unmistakable spherical structure with a prominent vagus nerve attached to its distal aspect. The nodose ganglion is clearly distinguished from the superior cervical sympathetic ganglion (first visible at E13) which is an elongated structure that is attached caudally to the sympathetic chain which is much thinner than the vagus nerve.

3. Dissociation of dissected neural tissue

Dissected neural tissue is incubated with trypsin, washed, and triturated to give a single cell suspension. The procedure is similar for mammalian and avian tissue of all embryonic stages, but the strength of the trypsin and incubation times need to be adjusted for the particular tissue.

Protocol 10. Preparation of neural single cell suspension

1. Use a Pasteur pipette to transfer the dissected tissue to a 10 ml conical tube containing 1–2 ml of Ca^{2+}/Mg^{2+}-free, Hank's balanced salt solution (CMF-HBSS). Wash the tissue by agitation and remove the CMF-HBSS. For chicken ganglia add 0.9 ml of fresh CMF-HBSS and 0.1 ml of 1% trypsin (Worthington) in CMF-HBSS (stored in aliquots at –20 °C). For mouse ganglia add 0.95 ml of fresh CMF-HBSS and 0.05 ml of 1% trypsin.

2. Immerse the lower end of the tube in a water-bath at 37 °C for 10 min

Protocol 10. *Continued*

for early sensory ganglia from chicken embryos, 15–20 min for mid-embryonic ganglia from chicken embryos, 5 min for early sensory ganglia from mouse embryos, and up to 10 min for older embryonic mouse sensory ganglia. These times are only a rough guide. They may need to be adjusted for different batches of trypsin. The optimum time is a compromise between neuronal damage due to over-trypsinization and neuronal damage due to vigorous trituration required to dissociate under-trypsinized tissue. If the tissue starts to disaggregate before trituration, the time is too long. If the tissue dissociates with difficulty and incompletely with trituration, the time is not long enough.

3. After trypsinization, remove most of the trypsin solution with a Pasteur pipette. Wash the tissue with 2 x 10 ml of Ham's F-12 or F-14 medium containing 10% heat activated horse serum to remove and inactivate residual trypsin. Removal of the medium is facilitated by pelleting the tissue between washings in a bench-top centrifuge at 2000 g for 1–2 min (this is essential for small ganglia). If the neurons are to be separated from the non-neuronal cells by differential sedimentation, it will be necessary to wash the tissue with about 5 ml of HBSS to remove traces of serum.

4. After washing, the tissue is dissociated into a single cell suspension by trituration. This is the most critical step. Use a siliconized Pasteur pipette. Heat the tip of the pipette in a Bunsen burner flame to form a fine bore. Triturate the tissue in culture medium if the cells are to be plated directly, or in HBSS without serum if the neurons are to be separated from non-neuronal cells by differential sedimentation. Use about 1.5 ml of medium or HBSS and take the tissue into the pipette and slowly expel the contents with firm pressure. If done correctly, the early ganglionic tissue should completely dissociate after three to five passages. In the case of older tissue, some connective tissue fragments may be left even after all of the neurons have dissociated. It is a mistake to carry on triturating older ganglia until all tissue fragments have dissociated. In the case of older ganglia, allow larger tissue fragments to settle after the first two to three passages, take the supernatant suspension into a fresh tube, and continue gentle trituration. Avoid over-trituration as this causes substantial neuronal damage, especially in the case of large, older neurons. Also avoid bubbles during trituration. Monitor the trituration by examining a drop of the dissociated cell suspension on a glass slide using an inverted phase-contrast microscope. A sensitive feature of over-zealous trituation is the loss of neuronal processes; neurons should still have fairly long processes attached to their cell bodies.

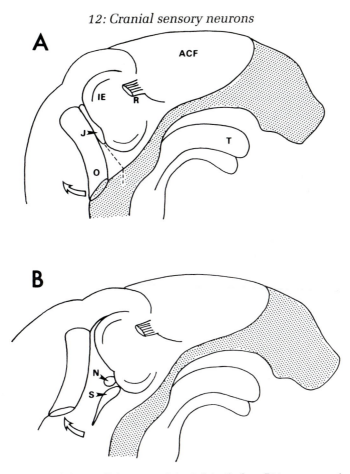

Figure 9. Drawings of the medial aspect of the left half of an E14 mouse embryo head showing successive stages in the dissection of the nodose ganglion. The bisected mid-line structures lying along and in front of the cranial base are stippled. (A) The incision passing from the jugular foramen (J) to the midline is shown by the interrupted line. The direction in which the large ossified part of the occipital bone (O) should be reflected to open up the jugular foramen after making the previous incision is shown by the large curved arrow. T, tongue; ACF, anterior cranial fossa; R, root of the trigeminal nerve; IE, inner ear. (B) The nodose ganglion (N) and superior cervical sympathetic ganglion (S) are revealed after extending the jugular foramen to the midline and reflecting the large ossified part of the occipital bone backwards.

It may be necessary to modify the above standard method in several ways:

(a) For large quantities of tissue, the release of DNA from disrupted cells can present difficulties in washing and trituration. This can be alleviated by the inclusion of bovine pancreatic DNase (Sigma, type IV) at a concentration of 40 µg/ml, plus 3 mM magnesium sulfate in the first HBSS/horse serum wash after trypsinization. Let the tissue sit in the solution at room temperature for about 5 min before washing again in HBSS/horse serum and proceeding as above.

(b) Because of the increasing amounts of collagenous connective tissue in late embryonic and more mature ganglia, this tissue may require treatment with collagenase prior to trypsinization. Use 500 μg/ml collagenase (Worthington) in F-12 for 10–15 min at 37 °C. Wash in HBSS before proceeding with the trypsinization.

4. Separation of neurons from non-neuronal cells

Because a variety of non-neuronal cells synthesize and release neurotrophic factors in culture, it is desirable to remove these cells prior to culture if one wishes to study the effects of neurotrophic factors on neurons. If they are not removed, the percentage neuronal survival in control cultures may be un-acceptably high. Furthermore, if non-neuronal cells are present, one cannot conclude that the effect of a factor or reagent on neuronal survival or some aspect of neuronal development or function is due to a direct action of the factor or reagent on neurons, or is mediated via the non-neuronal cells.

Two methods may be used to remove satellite cells and Schwann cells from mid to late embryonic dissociated ganglionic tissue: differential adhesion and differential sedimentation. Of the two, the method of differential sedimentation described here is more effective, reliable, and faster. It also avoids the problem of neuronal aggregation frequently encountered with differential adhesion and effectively removes all cellular debris. Differential adhesion does, however, have an advantage when the size difference between neurons and non-neuronal cells is very small (as in the case of the vestibular ganglion), and may be desirable in these instances. Neither method works well for very early ganglia which contain progenitor cells in addition to satellite and Schwann cells. In these cases the potential effects of factors produced by non-neuronal cells can be reduced by setting-up very low density cultures in a relatively large volume of culture medium (which is in anycase standard practice for older embryonic cultures) or by setting-up single cell cultures (14).

A further complication of early ganglionic cell cultures is that progenitor cells may differentiate into neurons in culture. Thus, in studying the effects of factors on the survival of early neurons one must bear in mind that an increase in the number neurons in early ganglionic cell cultures could result not only from the enhanced survival of differentiated neurons, but from enhanced rate of the differentiation of neurons from progenitor cells, or from an increase in progenitor cell proliferation which creates a large pool of pro-genitor cells that can subsequently differentiate into neurons. To distinguish between these alternatives it is necessary to follow the fates of individual neurons in these cultures (6).

4.1 Differential adhesion

This technique relies on the preferential adherence of non-neuronal cells to tissue culture plastic. The details described here are modified from the method described by Burnham and colleagues (15).

Protocol 11. Differential adhesion of neuronal cells

1. Dissociate the ganglia in culture medium (usually, F-14 plus 10% heat inactivated horse serum for embryonic chicken neurons).

2. Pre-plate this cell suspension in a total volume of 5 ml of medium plus 10% heat inactivated horse serum in a 90 mm tissue culture plastic Petri dish (Gibco BRL).

3. Place this in a humidified CO_2 incubator at 37 °C for 3–4 h. Remove the dish from the incubator toward the end of this period and monitor the attachment of cells with an inverted phase-contrast microscope. Discontinue pre-plating when almost all non-neuronal cells have attached.

4. Incline the dish at an angle and gently wash the surface of the dish with its contained medium using a Pasteur pipette to detach the loosely attached neurons. A variable number of neurons will remain attached to the dish, but do not attempt to detach these as vigorous washing will also detach non-neuronal cells.

4.2 Gravity sedimentation

This is without doubt the best technique. It depends on differences in sedimentation rates of cells in a liquid medium. Generally, the larger the cell, the faster its rate of sedimentation. Hence, neurons sediment more quickly than non-neuronal cells. Several variations of the method described by Miller and Phillips (16) have been applied to embryonic neural tissue (17–21). In contrast to these methods, the one described here is particularly easy to set-up as it requires neither specialized apparatus nor the establishment of density gradients. It is applicable to all populations of neurons in the peripheral nervous system and is very efficient (at least 60% of the neurons in the starting tissue are recovered uncontaminated by other cells). Furthermore, since the cells sediment through culture medium, neuronal viability is very high.

Protocol 12. Gravity sedimentation of neuronal cells

1. Sedimentation is carried out in a 100 ml cylindrical, siliconized, glass dropping funnel with a ground glass outlet tap (*Figure 10a*). Autoclave the funnel and its tap separately; place separate pieces of aluminium

---

Protocol 12. *Continued*

foil on the top, spout, and tap region before autoclaving. After assembly, fill the funnel to a height of 8–10 cm with F-14 medium plus 10% heat inactivated horse serum (thoroughly mixed and filtered through a 0.2 µm Millipore filter beforehand). Clamp the funnel vertically in a stand. Place this on a vibration-free surface in the cold (2 ± 0.5 °C) and leave overnight. I use a refrigerated incubator containing an anti-vibration table made from a concrete slab mounted on tennis balls.

2. Make up the dissociated cell suspension to a volume of about 2 ml in HBSS. Carefully layer the cell suspension on the medium by running it down the inside of the funnel and replace the foil top on the dropping funnel.

3. After an hour, remove the foil from the spout and run off 4–5 ml aliquots into sterile tubes.

4. Place 0.5 ml samples of these fractions in a 24-multiwell plate (16 mm diameter wells) and examine with phase-contrast microscopy to determine which fractions contain only neurons. Mid-embryonic and older neurons are clearly distinguished from other cells by their characteristic morphology (*Figure 10b*).

5. Pool the neuronal fractions and plate the neurons as described below.

It is not essential to have a refrigerated incubator to use this technique. The dropping funnel can be assembled, loaded, and drained in a cold room. Although the risk of bacterial and fungal contamination is greater, I have not experienced problems under these conditions. The technique works well between temperatures of 1–5 °C, although 2 °C is best. It is important to keep the temperature constant to avoid convection currents in this medium.

5. Culturing isolated neurons

5.1 Culture substratum

Neurons are grown on a laminin/polyornithine substratum. For most purposes, 35 mm diameter plastic tissue culture Petri dishes are used (in my experience, NUNC dishes available from Gibco BRL provide the best results). The substratum is prepared as detailed in *Protocol 13*.

Protocol 13. Preparation of the culture substratum

1. Place 1 ml of 0.5 mg/ml poly-DL-ornithine (P-8638, Sigma) in a 0.15 M borate buffer (pH 8.6) in each dish and let this stand overnight at room temperature. The poly-DL-ornithine solution should be filter

sterilized using a 0.2 μm filter and may be stored in glass bottles at 4 °C for up to two weeks.

2. Aspirate the polyornithine solution the following morning and wash the dishes three times with sterile distilled water. Let the dishes air dry in a laminar flow hood. Although the dried dishes should usually be coated with laminin and used the same day, they can be stored for at least a week at room temperature prior to coating with laminin.

3. Place 150 μl of a 20 μg/ml solution of laminin in F-14 medium in the centre of each dish and use the pipette tip to spread this over about two-thirds of the dish surface. Place the dishes in a culture incubator for at least 4 h. Laminin (Gibco) is available as a sterile solution. This should be thawed at 4 °C and aliquoted into sterile Eppendorf tubes. Store these at −70 °C until required. Thaw the required number of aliquots at 4 °C and dilute the laminin in F-14 immediately before use.

4. Remove the dishes from the incubator and wash the dishes twice with culture medium. Do not allow the dishes to dry between washes and place 1 ml of medium in each dish after washing. It is best to use the dishes straight after preparation, but they can be stored in the incubator with medium for up to two days but no longer.

5.2 Preparation of the culture medium

The best culture medium for embryonic neurons of the peripheral nervous system is F-14 (special formulation from Gibco). Powered F-14 should be made up with water of the highest purity. I routinely use water that has been sequentially passed through a charcoal filter, reverse osmosis system, and a Milli-Q system before being double distilled. Because F-14 should not be stored longer than three weeks in the refrigerator, it is convenient to make up a 10 × concentrate of F-14 (without added sodium bicarbonate, otherwise a precipitate will form) and store this in frozen 50 ml aliquots (kept at −20 °C or less). To make 1 × F-14, add 1 g of sodium bicarbonate to 450 ml of water, then add a 50 ml aliquot of 10 × F-14 and bubble CO_2 through the medium until the pH reaches between pH 6.5 and pH 7 (I find the medium stores better at a slightly more acid pH than the physiological optimum of pH 7.2–7.4). The medium should then be filter sterilized and stored at 4 °C. It is vital that all glassware is thoroughly clean and free of any traces of detergent.

For culturing embryonic chicken neurons, the medium should be supplemented with 10% heat inactivated horse serum that should always be filtered through a 0.2 μm filter before use. In my experience, serum obtained from Gibco gives the best results. For embryonic mouse neurons, serum is best avoided. Instead the following supplements should be added to the medium: 2 mM glutamine, 0.35% bovine serum albumin (Pathocyte-4, ICN), 60 ng/ml progesterone, 16 μg/ml putrescine, 400 ng/ml L-thyroxine, 38 ng/ml sodium

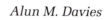

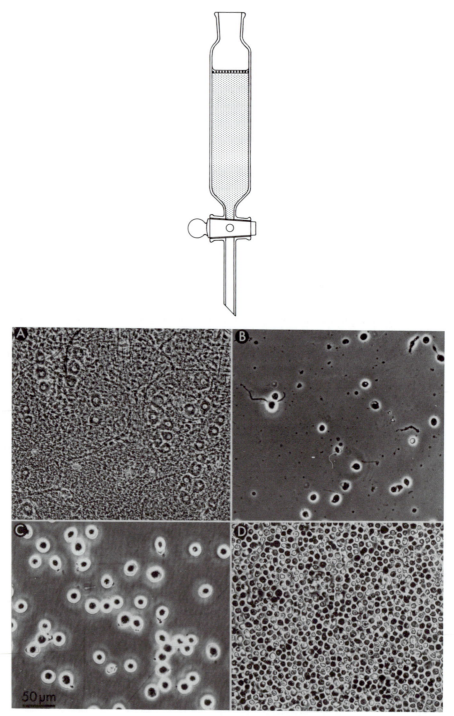

Figure 10. (a) Drawing of a dropping funnel showing a cell suspension (heavy stipple) layered on culture medium (light stipple). (b) Phase-contrast micrographs showing the successive stages in the separation of TMN neurons from other cells by differential sedimentation. (A) The intact median part of the TMN showing several TMN neurons (*arrows*). (B) Dissociated cell suspension showing a single neuron (*arrow*), numerous non-neuronal cells, and cellular debris. (C) An aliquot of neuronal cells taken from the dropping funnel after sedimentation (neuronal processes largely retract into the cell body during sedimentation). (D) An aliquot of non-neuronal cells taken from the dropping funnel after sedimentation. From ref. 13.

---

selenite, and 340 ng/ml triiodothyronine. For convenience, these additives are combined to make a 50 × concentrate that is stored in 10 ml aliquots at −20 °C.

5.3 Seeding the neurons

To carry out, for example, a dose response to a neurotrophic factor, first set-up a suitable range of dilutions in culture medium at double the required final concentration. Remove the culture medium from the washed Petri dishes and place 1 ml of each dilution in triplicate dishes. Control dishes (at least four) should each receive 1 ml of medium. To avoid possible observer bias, code the dishes.

For the best results, the neurons should be plated at a density of between 500 and 2000 per dish. Place the suspension of neurons in a suitable volume of medium in a large screw-top tube (e.g. 50 ml centrifuge tube) and evenly distribute the neurons in the medium by gently rocking the tube end-over-end several times. Distribute the neurons to the dishes using a microlitre pipette in two lots of 0.5 ml (to further ensure even distribution). Avoid touching the medium in the dishes with the pipette tip, otherwise small quantities of neurotrophic factor will be transferred to other dishes. Return the dishes to a humidified CO_2 incubator at 37 °C (use 4% CO_2 for F-14 medium). Because of the very low neuron density required, the most reliable method of estimating the correct neuron density at the time of plating neurons is by eye. Place 1 ml of the cell suspension in a test culture dish and examine the resulting neuron suspension with a phase-contrast microscope. Experience will guide the necessary adjustments that may need to be made to the number of neurons in the cell suspension.

5.4 Neuronal survival

A standard graticule for examining the same area of each culture dish is required. This is made from the base of a 900 mm plastic Petri dish using a scalpel blade to inscribe a 12 x 12 mm square divided into 2 mm squares (using graph paper as a template).

Protocol 14. Quantification of neuronal survival

1. Mount the graticule on the stage of an inverted phase-contrast microscope with the inscribed surface uppermost.

2. Determine the number of neurons seeded per dish by examining several dishes after 6 h in culture. Centre each dish over the graticule and count the number of neurons within the inscribed area (scan each row of 2 mm squares in turn). A small percentage of neurons (usually less than 10%) will have been damaged during dissociation and will not attach to the substratum. I usually ignore these neurons and only count those that have attached.

3. Count the number of surviving neurons in all dishes after at least 48 h in culture. In almost all cases, long neurites will have grown from these neurons.

4. The survival response of neurons to a particular neurotrophic factor is conveniently expressed as percentage survival: the quotient of the number of attached neurons in the graticule area at 6 h and the number surviving at in this same area at 48 h expressed as a percentage.

Acknowledgements

Research in my laboratory is supported by grants from The Wellcome Trust, Medical Research Council, Cancer Research Campaign, Action Research, Science and Engineering Research Council, and The Royal Society.

References

1. Davies, A. M. (1989). *Nature*, **337**, 553.
2. Vogel, K. S. and Davies, A. M. (1993). *Development*, **119**, 263.
3. Lumsden, A. G. and Davies, A. M. (1983). *Nature*, **306**, 786.
4. Lumsden, A. G. and Davies, A. M. (1986). *Nature*, **323**, 538.
5. Davies, A. M., Bandtlow, C., Heumann, R., Korsching, S., Rohrer, H., and Thoenen, H. (1987). *Nature*, **326**, 353.
6. Buchman, V. I. and Davies, A. M. (1993). *Development*, **118**, 989.
7. Davies, A. M., Thoenen, H., and Barde, Y. A. (1986). *Nature*, **319**, 497.
8. Allsopp, T., Wyatt, S., Patterson, H., and Davies, A. M. (1993). *Cell*, **73**, 295.
9. Allsopp, T., Robinson, M., Wyatt, S., and Davies, A. M. (1993). *J. Cell Biol.*, **123**, 1555–66.
10. Hamburger, V. and Hamilton, H. L. (1951). *J. Morphol.*, **88**, 49.
11. Davies, A. M. and Lindsay, R. M. (1985). *Dev. Biol.*, **111**, 62.
12. Davies, A. M., Thoenen, H., and Barde, Y.-A. (1986). *J. Neurosci.*, **6**, 1897.
13. Davies, A. M. (1986). *Dev. Biol.*, **115**, 56.

14. Wright, E., Vogel, K. S., and Davies, A. M. (1992). *Neuron*, **9,** 139.
15. Burnham, P., Raiborn, C., and Varon, S. (1972). *Proc. Natl. Acad. Sci. USA*, **69,** 3556.
16. Miller, R. G. and Phillips, R. A. (1969). *J. Cell Physiol.*, **73,** 191.
17. Lam, D. M. K. (1972). *Proc. Natl. Acad. Sci. USA*, **69,** 1987.
18. Barkley, D. S., Rakic, L., Chaffe, J. D., and Wong, D. L. (1973). *J. Cell Physiol.*, **81,** 271.
19. Cohen, J., Balazs, R., Hajos, F., Currie, D. N., and Dutton, G. R. (1978). *Brain Res.*, **148,** 313.
20. Cohen, J., Mares, V., and Lodin, Z. (1973). *J. Neurochem.*, **20,** 651.
21. Berg, D. K. and Fischbach, G. D. (1978). *J. Cell Biol.*, **77,** 83.
22. Davies, A. M. (1988). *IBRO Handbook*, **12,** 95.
23. Davies, A. M. and Lumsden, A. G. S. (1984). *J. Comp. Neurol.*, **223,** 124.

13

Avian ciliary and lumbar sympathetic ganglion neurons

RAE NISHI

1. Introduction

Chick parasympathetic and sympathetic ganglia provide a convenient source of readily isolated and cultured neurons that have a variety of uses:

- bioassays for trophic factors by quantifying survival of neurons in response to defined or undefined activities
- bioassays for neurite outgrowth promoting activities
- bioassays for neurotransmitter plasticity

In particular, the chick ciliary ganglion is a relatively homogeneous source of cholinergic parasympathetic neurons that innervates striated muscle very readily, hence it has been invaluable for studies of molecular changes associated with neuromuscular synapse formation.

The relative success of preparing primary neuronal cultures depends on a number of variables, not just how the dissection and dissociation are done. As a result, I have included detailed protocols and discussion of each of what I view to be the most important considerations when making cultures. Clearly, each variable must be optimized for the use to which you expect to apply your cultures. That is, set-up your cultures and test them for whatever your assay will be, and make sure each variable is optimized for what you want to see. Thus, those studies that require long-term cultures that follow transmitter phenotype or synapse formation will require more stringent conditions and stricter adherence to protocol than studies that merely want to quantify neuronal survival or process outgrowth after 24 hours in culture. If you want the best, most reproducible results, my advice is to be extremely rigorous in your adherence to the protocols, and do not allow 'slop' in measurements or times of incubation.

2. Dissection of ciliary and lumbar sympathetic ganglia

2.1 Comments

As soon as the organism is killed anoxia initiates a number of degenerative processes which can be minimized if the solutions in which the tissues are bathed are kept cold and if the ganglia of interest are isolated free from other tissue as rapidly as possible. Embryonic tissues are extremely fragile and soft with little colour contrast for identifying structures, thus it is often helpful to immerse them completely in isotonic saline to buoy the structures and preserve morphology. The saline used for dissection should contain calcium and magnesium to preserve tissue integrity, glucose to provide an energy source, and it should not be buffered with bicarbonate because the pH will become rapidly alkaline if left at atmospheric CO_2 concentrations for extended periods of time. Optimal contrast in identifying embryonic structures is also obtained by using a dissection microscope with indirect transillumination. To prevent sticking of tissues to dissecting instruments the instruments should be very clean and free of debris.

2.2 Suggested age of embryos to use for dissections

2.2.1 Ciliary ganglia

Ciliary ganglia are most readily dissected and cultured if removed from embryonic day 7.5–8 chickens (Hamburger-Hamilton Stage 34). At this stage the chicks do not yet have pin feathers and two-thirds to all of the scleral papillae have formed around the eye. This is prior to the time of cell death in the ganglion, so more neurons can be recovered. After this time the number of non-neuronal cells in the ganglion increases dramatically, thus resulting in greater contamination of the neuronal cultures with fibroblasts and satellite cells.

2.2.2 Lumbar sympathetic ganglia

The lumbar sympathetic ganglia are most readily found and dissected after embryonic day 12. Although one can identify the ganglia at earlier stages the population is mixed in that it contains both differentiating neuroblasts and postmitotic neurons. After embryonic day 13 the ganglia become increasingly difficult to dissociate with trypsin and contain increasingly more non-neuronal cells.

Protocol 1. Dissection of ciliary ganglia

Equipment and reagents

- One straight, blunt-ended 4–6 inch long forceps
- One curved, blunt-ended 4–6 inch long forceps
- Two Dumont No. 5 forceps
- Two No. 2 iridectomy knives
- One straight, 3 inch long scissors (for sympathetic dissection only)
- Two 100 x 20 mm sterile glass Petri dishes
- One 60 x 15 mm sterile glass Petri dish
- Sterile Hepes-buffered Earle's balanced salt solution (EBSS)
- Sterile modified Puck's solution with glucose (MPG)
- Sterile, cotton plugged 9 inch Pasteur pipettes
- Sterile 15 ml polystyrene conical centrifuge tube with cap
- Chicken eggs: preferably 8 days of incubation (E8) for ciliary ganglia, and E13 for sympathetic ganglia
- Low power dissecting microscope (x 3–70 magnification) that can illuminate preparation from above or below

Method

1. Sterilize the instruments in 70% ethanol for at least 20 min.

2. Squirt each egg twice with 70% ethanol (allow ethanol to dry between applications).

3. Crack the egg and pull the shell off with the straight, blunt forceps; remove the embryo with the curved forceps by hooking them around the neck.

4. Place embryo into 100 mm Petri dish that is about two-thirds full of cold EBSS; remove all embryos at once.

5. Using the curved forceps, cut the heads off by pinching the neck between the forceps tips; transfer the heads to the second 100 mm dish containing EBSS. Place dish with heads on stage of dissecting microscope with the light coming from above; position 60 mm Petri dish containing 10 ml of cold MPG near the microscope with the lid off.

6. Using the Dumont No. 5 forceps, position the head with the beak pointing up. Hold the head down with one pair of forceps pinned in the neck and use the other pair to pinch through the skin and extraocular tissue around the orbit of the eye. Work about three-quarters of the way around, pinching and cutting through the skin and muscle, but not piercing the eye (*Figure 1A*).

7. Place one pair of forceps in the orbit of the eye against the beak; place the other pair of forceps against the eye and gently rotate the eye away from the orbit. Look for the optic nerve. Just below the optic nerve you will see a ganglion suspended by its pre- and post-ganglionic nerve. That is the ciliary ganglion. Keep rotating the eye until the optic nerve breaks (*Figure 1B*).

8. Turn the loose eyeball over so you can see the optic nerve and the

Protocol 1. *Continued*

choroid fissure. The ciliary ganglion should be between the optic nerve and the fissure. It is small, white, and round. Often, you will see a nerve attached (*Figure 1C*).

9. Remove the ganglion by grabbing the postganglionic nerve (the one that attaches the ganglion to the eye); transfer the ganglion to the 60 mm Petri dish.

10. After you have collected all the ganglia you want, position the 60 mm dish with the ganglia under the scope, switch the light from above to below (i.e. transilluminate the ganglia), increase the magnification (to about x 10).

11. Using your forceps, push all the ganglia down below the surface tension of the solution so they sink to the bottom (many of the ganglia will be floating). Collect all the submerged ganglia together in the centre of the dish by gently swirling the dish.

12. Using the iridectomy knives in a 'scissoring' action, trim the extra mesodermal tissue off the ganglia and cut the nerves as close as possible to the ganglion. This will minimize non-neuronal contamination of the cell culture. Once the ganglia have been cleaned, push them to a different part of the dish and count them.

13. Remove the ganglia with a pre-wetted 9 inch Pasteur pipette (don't suck the ganglia past where the tip enlarges, or they will get stuck when you try to blow them out); transfer ganglia to sterile 15 ml conical centrifuge tube.

Protocol 2. Dissection of lumbar sympathetic ganglia

1. Remove E13 embryo from egg as described above and transfer to dry 100 mm Petri dish. Immediately cut head off with sterile scissors.

2. Turn body back side up and cut along the outside of the spinal column to remove the strip of body wall that contains the lumbar spinal column (*Figure 2A*).

3. Transfer strip of spinal column/cord to a Petri dish filled with saline and clean the internal face free of organ parts and blood vessels using a stereoscope with light coming from above the preparation.

4. Transfer cleaned strip to 60 mm dish containing 10 ml sterile MPG (*Figure 2B*). Turn strip so that internal face is toward the light—you will see the outline of the spinal column and alongside, the sympathetic chain—run an iridectomy knife blade along the outside of the sympathetic chain to cut the postganglionic nerves (*Figure 2C*).

5. Grasp the sympathetic column at one end with a pair of Dumont No. 5 forceps and pull up as you use an iridectomy knife to cut the preganglionic nerves to the sympathetic chain (*Figure 2D*). Set the chain down in the bottom of the same dish; discard the spinal column once all the sympathetic ganglia that you can see have been removed.

6. Using the iridectomy knives, cut the ganglia free from the chain, cutting the connectives as close to the ganglion as possible. With transillumination the ganglia can be readily distinguished from connectives by the texture (ganglia contain round, spherical dots, while connectives look like bundles of cables).

7. Count the number of ganglia you have, then carefully transfer them to a sterile conical centrifuge tube with a pre-wetted Pasteur pipette.

3. Dissociation of ganglia

3.1 Comments

The following protocol works very well for many different types of ganglia isolated from chicken embryos. Optimal yields of viable neurons are obtained when one is extremely careful about trypsinization and mechanical dissociation. Trypsin is a very potent protease that works well to dissociate tissue, but if digestion conditions are not carefully controlled, trypsin can reduce neuronal viability. Trypsin lots can be very variable, even when purchased from the same source. We routinely purchase 2.5% sterile trypsin solution from Gibco-BRL and have found that anywhere from 0.06% to 0.125% works best in digesting ganglia without reducing viability.

The strength of mechanical dissociation used can also cause cell damage. The opening of the Pasteur pipette to be used to triturate the ganglia should be fire-polished and reduced in diameter by about one-half. When triturating, care should be taken to minimize air introduction (bubbling), which will lyse cells. I often count the number of times I must pipette the ganglia up and down in the Pasteur pipette before they become completely dissociated. If they dissociate in 30 trips up and down, then the trypsinization or the strength of trituration (i.e. the bore of the pipette or the speed that you are triturating) is too much, and many cells will be damaged. If it takes 40–90 times, then its about right. If it takes more than 100 times, then the trypsin is too weak or you haven't closed the bore of the pipette down enough. The greatest consistency in plating will be achieved if incubation times and the process of trituration is adhered to most closely.

1

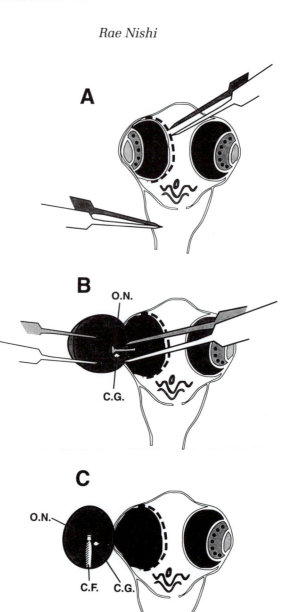

Figure 1. Dissection of the ciliary ganglion. (A) View of E8 chicken head with beak facing up showing where to cut around orbit of eye. (B) View of head as eye is being rotated out. Optic nerve (O.N.) is still attached to the brain but stretched; similarly, the ciliary ganglion (C.G.) is still attached by its preganglionic nerve. (C) View of head after eye is completely rotated out and both optic nerve and preganglionic ciliary ganglion nerve have snapped. The ciliary ganglion can be seen as a small round object just inferior and medial to the stump of the optic nerve. The choroid fissure (C.F.) can be clearly seen lateral to the ganglion.

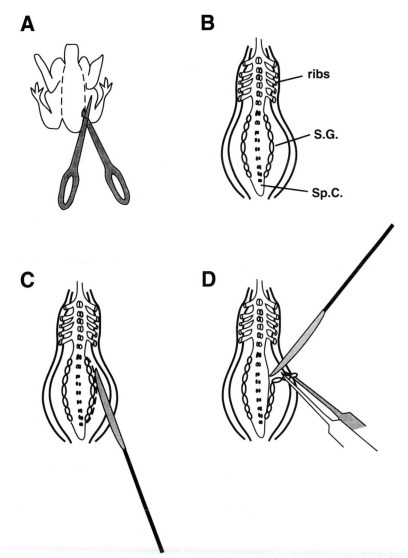

A

B

ribs

S.G.

Sp.C.

C

D

Figure 2. Dissection of the lumbar sympathetic ganglia. (A) Embryo with backside up showing where to cut around the spinal column with a pair of scissors. (B) View of dissected body wall with spinal column (Sp.C.) lying ventral side up and with all organs removed. The sympathetic ganglia (S.G.) can be seen along the side of the spinal column. Ganglia are drawn larger than actual size. (C) Location of first cut outside of sympathetic chain to sever postganglionic nerves. (D) How to remove sympathetic chain with forceps while cutting preganglionic nerves.

Protocol 3. Dissociation of ganglia

Equipment and reagents

- 15 ml polystyrene conical centrifuge tube containing dissected and cleaned ganglia (see above)
- Sterile MPG (see *Protocol 1*)
- Complete medium with 10% heat inactivated horse serum (see section 4.2)
- Sterile 2.5% trypsin (Gibco-BRL)
- Sterile 9 inch Pasteur pipettes with cotton plugs
- Amber latex Pasteur pipette bulb
- Water-bath set at 37 °C
- Table-top clinical centrifuge

Method

1. Add 2.4 ml MPG to the centrifuge tube containing the ganglia. Add 0.1 ml 2.5% trypsin to the MPG (final trypsin concentration is 0.1%) and gently agitate the tube to mix the trypsin into the solution.

2. Incubate ganglia at 37 °C in a water-bath for 20 min.

3. Spin ganglia down to bottom of tube at 200–250 *g*. Carefully remove the supernatant with a Pasteur pipette. Add 3 ml complete medium with serum.

4. Attach amber bulb to sterile Pasteur pipette and flame opening until the diameter is reduced by about one-half. Do not pull pipette tip out further after heating the glass; do not use larger bulb, or pipette aid, or any other pipetting device.

5. Gently triturate ganglia (pipette ganglia up and down). Do not introduce air into the solution or you will create many bubbles that will lyse cells. Watch ganglia while triturating; stop when you can no longer see bits of tissue. The ganglia will have to be moved up and down the Pasteur pipette about 50 to 100 times before they are completely dissociated.

6. Spin cells down in clinical centrifuge at 200–250 *g* for 5 min. Remove supernatant with Pasteur pipette. (Don't use an aspirator or you will accidentally suck out the cells.)

7. Resuspend cells at a concentration of one ciliary ganglion equivalent per 0.1 ml (e.g. if you collected 40 ganglia, resuspend them in 4 ml) of complete medium, or resuspend sympathetic ganglia in a known volume of medium (e.g. 2 ml) and count cells on a haemocytometer. Plate neurons at densities of about 8000–9000 neurons/cm^2 (for ciliary ganglia this is equivalent to one ganglion per each well of a 24-well plate where the diameter is approx. 1 cm).

4. Culturing ciliary and sympathetic ganglia

4.1 Comments

One day after plating all of the viable neurons should be attached directly to the substratum and not merely on top of non-neuronal cells. Cellular debris should be minimal. The cell bodies should look smooth and phase-bright, and many neurites should already have initiated and extended several cell body diameters (*Figure 3*).

Poor attachment and stunted neurite outgrowth indicate that the substratum or the medium supplementation (presence of appropriate trophic factors) is not optimal; rough, phase-dark cell bodies with a large amount of cellular debris indicate that the dissociation was too rough.

Cultures that survive the first 48 hours after plating can usually be maintained for many days, provided that trophic factors are replenished by feeding and that no toxic substances are inadvertently introduced (see below).

4.2 Medium

Basic medium that we use for both ciliary and lumbar sympthetic ganglia is Eagles minimal essential medium supplemented with 50 U/ml penicillin, 50 µg/ml streptomycin, 2 mM glutamine, and 10% (v/v) heat inactivated horse serum. The penicillin, streptomycin, and glutamine can be purchased as sterile 100 x stock solutions from commercial vendors (e.g. Gibco-BRL, Microbiological Associates, Sigma). Sera available for cell culture tend to be very variable and differ greatly in their quality, therefore we pre-test different lots of horse serum from several different vendors for their ability to support long-term (10–14 days) ciliary ganglion cell survival in the presence of ciliary neurotrophic factor (CNTF) or growth promoting activity (GPA), and then purchase a large quantity and store it at –20 °C. Serum that is already heat inactivated can be purchased from some vendors. If the serum you buy is not heat inactivated, then incubate a 100 ml bottle at 56 °C in a water-bath for 30 min, then spin at 40 000 g in a refrigerated centrifuge for 45 min to remove precipitated material.

Both ciliary ganglion and sympathetic neurons cannot survive in cell culture without the addition of neurotrophic factors. Although crude sources of trophic factors (e.g. 5% chick embryo extract) can be used, it is considerably more preferable to use a purified or recombinant trophic factor. Fortunately, a number of molecules that support sympathetic or ciliary ganglion survival have now been identified (see *Table 1*). With the exception of growth promoting activity (GPA) all of the trophic factors listed below are now commercially available from companies such as Collaborative Research, Upstate Biotechnology, Inc., Gibco-BRL, and Sigma). Obviously, the choice of any particular one for your cell culture system may have significant impact on the outcome of your experiment. An essential fact to keep in mind is that many

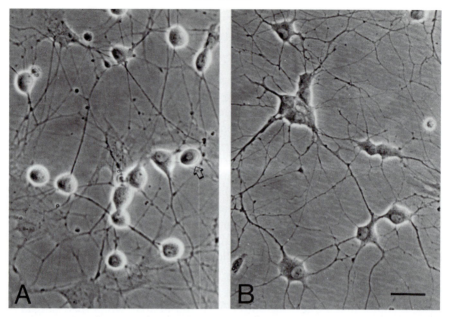

Figure 3. Phase-contrast photographs of cultures 24 hours after plating. (A) Ciliary ganglion neurons. E8 ciliary ganglia were dissociated and plated on polylysine/laminin in complete medium (see text) containing 20 ng/ml CNTF. Open arrow indicates a red blood cell. (B) Lumbar sympathetic neurons. E13 lumbar sympathetic ganglia were dissociated and plated as described above. Photographs were made using a x 25 water-immersion lens with phase-contrast optics. Calibration bar equals 20 μm.

trophic factors are very labile, and hence, cannot be kept for very long once they have been diluted into complete medium. We always aliquot trophic factors into one-time use volumes and store them at –80 °C (long-term storage) or at –20 °C (e.g. short-term storage between feedings). The factors are thawed and added to the culture medium just prior to feeding.

Chick embryo eye extract (1%) is still often used as a source of trophic support for ciliary ganglion neurons (5). A number of scientists have since contacted me to report that their ciliary ganglion neuron cultures look beautiful in eye extract for the first three to four days, then suddenly die four to seven days after plating. We have also noted that this can occur with eye extract if excessively large amounts of eye extract are used (> 50 mg/ml of total protein). There appears to be a contaminating activity that causes healthy ciliary ganglion neurons to suddenly lyse and die after four to seven days in culture. We have found that this activity behaves as a macromolecule, and have even identified peaks of this activity from both gel sizing and chromatofocusing columns (Nishi, unpublished results). This molecule has yet to be isolated and the mechanism by which it causes death after such a pro-

Table 1. Molecules that support the survival of ciliary and sympathetic ganglion neurons in cell culture

Molecule	Specificity	Linear concentration range	Saturating concentration
7s NGF (1)	Sympathetic only	0.1–0.5 µg/ml	> 1 µg/ml
2.5s NGF (2)	Sympathetic only	0.01–0.5 ng/ml	> 1 ng/ml
CNTF (3)	CG and sympathetic	0.1–1.0 ng/ml	> 1 ng/ml
GPA (4)	CG and sympathetic	1.0–10 pg/ml	> 0.1 ng/ml
aFGF (4)	CG and sympathetic	0.01–0.1 ng/ml	> 1 ng/ml
bFGF (4)	CG and sympathetic	0.01–0.1 ng/ml	> 1 ng/ml

longed period of exposure is not known. We have never observed this mysterious 'death activity' with recombinant trophic factor (CNTF, aFGF, or bFGF).

4.3 Reduction of the number of non-neuronal cells

A major concern in many types of neuronal culture systems is to reduce or eliminate the non-neuronal cells that can overgrow the neurons and mask the direct effects of environmental manipulations on neurons. Non-neuronal cell contamination is a problem if the dissection/dissociation procedure brings a large number of satellite cells and fibroblasts or if the medium contains molecules that are mitogenic to the non-neuronal cells.

The number of non-neuronal cells that are plated can be significantly reduced by using E7.5–8 ciliary and E12–13 sympathetic ganglia and by carefully cleaning the ganglia free of attached nerve and adherent meshenchymal tissue. The mitogenicity of the medium can be controlled by using horse serum instead of fetal calf serum and by using defined trophic factors to support neuronal survival rather than crude extracts.

In our experience, techniques such as pre-plating the cell suspension to deplete fibroblasts results in fewer neurons recovered; in addition, chick neurons appear to be considerably more sensitive to antimitotic agents such as cytosine arabinoside than rat or mouse neurons. If an antimitotic agent must be used, then use lower than suggested concentrations of cytosine arabinoside ($< 10^{-5}$ M) or use antimitotic agents that are less toxic (fluorodeoxyuridine plus uridine at 10^{-5} M). Bear in mind if you use antimitotic agents, that they only kill rapidly dividing cells such as fibroblasts and not more slowly dividing (or non-dividing) cells such as Schwann cells. Interestingly, the use of aFGF or bFGF in supporting ciliary or sympathetic neuron survival does not seem to induce proliferation of the ganglionic non-neuronal cells (R. Nishi, unpublished results).

References

1. Chun, L. L. Y. and Patterson, P. H. (1977). *J. Cell Biol.*, **75,** 694.
2. Greene, L. (1977). *Dev. Biol.*, **58,** 95.
3. McDonald, J. R., Ko., C., Mismer, D., Smith, D. J., and Collins, F. (1991). *Biochim. Biophys. Acta*, **1090,** 70.
4. Eckenstein, F. P., Esch, F., Holbert, T., Blacher, R. W., and Nishi, R. (1990). *Neuron*, **4,** 623.
5. Nishi, R. and Berg, D. K. (1981). *J. Neurosci.*, **1,** 505.

14

Enteric ganglion cells

M. JILL SAFFREY

1. Introduction

The enteric nervous system (ENS), the intrinsic nervous system of the gut, is the largest part of the peripheral nervous system (PNS) and is responsible for the co-ordination of intestinal functions. Intestinal reflexes occur largely independently of input from the central nervous system (CNS) or other parts of the PNS, hence the ENS is a highly complex system, containing several types of motoneurons, interneurons, and sensory neurons. This functional heterogeneity is reflected in the great diversity of neurotransmitters employed by enteric neurons (see ref. 1). The ENS also differs considerably from other parts of the PNS in its organization. Unlike other peripheral ganglia, enteric ganglia contain no connective tissue or blood vessels; a major part of enteric ganglia consists of synaptic neuropil. Enteric glial cells are also distinctive, but show a number of similarities to astrocytes. In terms of neuronal diversity, ganglion organization, ultrastructural features, and glial cell characteristics, the ganglia of the ENS have therefore been likened to the CNS (2,3).

The enteric neurons (of which there are some 10^8 in the guinea-pig) are grouped into two ganglionated plexuses. These plexuses are intramural; the myenteric plexus is embedded between the two outer muscle layers of the gut wall; the submucous plexus lies deeper in the gut, within the connective tissue of the submucosa. The plexuses are connected and extend for the entire length of the gastrointestinal tract and, in almost all areas, completely around the gut wall. The enteric ganglia vary greatly in size and shape, according to the region of the gut and species. Myenteric ganglia are larger than submucous plexus ganglia (e.g. on average, 43 neurons/ganglion compared to 8 neurons/ganglion in the guinea-pig ileum). Processes from enteric neurons project to all layers of the gut wall.

2. Problems in the isolation of intramural ganglia

Like other intramural ganglia, enteric ganglia are difficult to isolate and culture as pure nervous tissue (4). This is because, despite their large number, they are small and embedded within the tissue which they innervate. This has meant that, compared to sympathetic and sensory ganglia which can readily be obtained by dissection in their entirety and uncontaminated by other tissues, enteric ganglion cells have been relatively little studied in culture. Early studies employed explants of the entire gut wall or of the outer muscle layers and had the obvious disadvantage that the non-neural cells heavily outnumbered the enteric ganglion cells (4).

Unlike other intramural ganglia, however, enteric ganglia are distributed in a regular arrangement within the wall of the digestive tract. In addition, the laminar nature of the different tissue elements of the gut wall facilitates their separation. For example, the outer muscle layers containing the myenteric plexus can, at least in some parts of the gut of some species, be readily separated from the underlying submucosa and mucosa. More recent methods for the culture of enteric ganglion cells have taken advantage of these histological features of the gut.

A method for isolating intact enteric ganglia from the non-neural tissues of the intestine was developed some 15 years ago (5,6). This method uses a combination of enzyme digestion and microdissection techniques to separate groups of intact myenteric or submucous plexus ganglia from surrounding smooth muscle and connective tissue of the gut wall (see section 3). These ganglia can then be grown as explants (section 4) which contain both enteric neurons and glial cells, but not smooth muscle or other types of intestinal cells. The separated ganglia can also be dissociated into a cell suspension before culture (7) (see section 6). In addition, explant cultures of myenteric ganglia can be manipulated *in vitro* to produce enriched cultures of neurons or glial cells (8) (see section 5). The use of enteric ganglia which have been freed from the gut wall and which are uncontaminated by smooth muscle and other cell types has clear advantages for the study of the ENS in culture, and such preparations have been quite widely used (4). However, a disadvantage of this approach is that, in most cases, it is necessary to use postnatal animals, as embryonic enteric ganglia are difficult to isolate by microdissection. Nevertheless, this is the only method which allows study of pure preparations of enteric ganglion cells.

Alternative methods for the culture of enteric neurons involve the dissociation of the whole gut wall, or some of its constituent layers, into cell suspensions. These suspensions contain a mixture of cell types, which vary according to the starting material. In order to reduce the numbers of non-neural cells, the outer muscle layers have been used as starting material for myenteric neurons (9,10), and the submucosa for submucosal neurons (11). Although subsequent enrichment for neurons is routine in these methods, resulting cultures still contain significant numbers of non-neural cells, which hamper studies requiring pure cell populations and defined culture conditions. However, an advantage of this type of dissociation approach is that embryonic tissue can be used. More sophisticated cell separation techniques are also now available, allowing purer cell populations to be obtained. For example, immunoselection techniques have recently been developed which allow the separation of enteric ganglion cell precursors from embryonic gut (12). These mixed cell type dissociation methods will not be detailed here, but are given in the references cited above.

3. Dissection of intact enteric ganglia from the gut wall

Myenteric ganglia have been isolated from the small and large intestines of several rodents, including guinea-pigs, rabbits, and rats, and also from chicks. Submucous plexus ganglia have been isolated from the large intestines of new-born guinea-pigs.

Segments of the outer muscle layers (or the entire gut wall) are cut into small pieces and incubated in collagenase (see *Protocol 1*). Groups of interconnected ganglia are then isolated by removal of the surrounding smooth muscle by microdissection (see *Protocols 2* and *3*, and *Figure 1*). Collagenase is the main enzyme used—myenteric plexus from the neonatal guinea-pig and 14–21 day rat intestines can be isolated using this enzyme alone. Elastase, hyaluronidase, and/or trypsin, used together or sequentially with collagenase, may be more suitable for other species, or for particular areas or ages of tissue. Batches of enzyme vary and should be tested—increases or decreases in incubation time or changes in concentration may be necessary for optimum dissection.

Protocol 1. Preparation of collagenase solution

1. Make up a 2 mg/ml solution of collagenase in Hank's BSS.

2. Stir, on ice, for 30–60 min.

3. Filter through 0.22 μm Millipore filter.

4. Aliquot (1 ml for final working volume of 2 ml).

5. Store frozen at –20 °C.

3.1 Myenteric ganglia

Where possible, the outer muscle layers rather than the entire gut wall are used as starting material, to avoid the need for antibiotic treatment for decontamination from intestinal micro-organisms (see section 3.1.1). This is most easily achieved in the guinea-pig caecum, where the outer longitudinal muscle forms thick bands, or taenia coli (see *Figure 1*). Another advantage is that the myenteric plexus forms a more closely-packed, easily manipulated network, with a large number of neurons, in this area of the guinea-pig gut. It

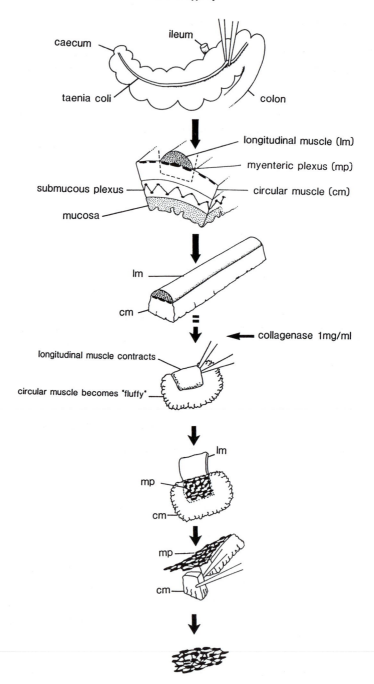

Figure 1. Dissection of myenteric plexus segments from beneath the taenia coli of the guinea-pig caecum (not to scale).

is recommended that, if possible, this tissue is used for practice in initial dissections.

The methods used for the isolating the myenteric plexus from the taenia coli and from other areas of the gut differ and are described separately below.

3.1.1 Myenteric ganglia from beneath the guinea-pig taenia coli

The procedure for isolation of myenteric ganglia from guinea-pig taenia coli is described in *Protocol 2* and shown diagrammatically in *Figure 1*. Neonatal guinea-pigs of between one and five-days-old have typically been used, but this method can be also be applied to older animals.

Protocol 2. Isolation of myenteric ganglia from beneath the guinea-pig taenia coli

Equipment and reagents

- Sterile dissecting instruments, including iridectomy (Vanna's) scissors and two pairs of fine watchmaker's forceps (No. 5)
- Dissecting microscope with oblique illumination (up to x 40 magnification—preferably in laminar flow hood)
- Balanced salt solution (BSS; Hank's BSS or similar)
- Collagenase solution (see *Protocol 1*)
- Concentrated antibiotic solution (if necessary, see text)
- Sterile 35 mm Petri dishes (or similar size)
- Sterile Pasteur pipettes
- Culture medium (medium 199 see section 4.1)

Method

All manipulations are best performed in a tissue culture cabinet.

1. Open the body cavity below the diaphragm aseptically, exposing the intestines.

2. Gently move the caecum to top.

3. Using dissecting microscope at x 10 magnification remove sections of the taenia coli, together with some underlying circular muscle (see *Figure 1*). This is best accomplished by holding the iridectomy scissors at a very acute angle (almost parallel) to the gut wall. If the caecum is pierced during this part of the dissection, releasing intestinal contents, remove segments of the entire gut wall, clean, and decontaminate these as described in section 3.1.1.

4. Cut the tissue into pieces of approx. 1 mm in length and place these into 1 mg/ml collagenase.

5. Either: place at 4°C overnight to allow penetration of enzyme, then incubate at 37°C for 20–60 min (according to the batch of enzyme), or incubate for 2–4 h at 37°C.

6. Using the dissecting microscope at x 20 magnification, gently remove

---

Protocol 2. *Continued*

smooth muscle with watchmaker's forceps, as shown in *Figure 1*. Take care to avoid touching the plexus with forceps—it is better to gently pull muscle against muscle. The outer, longitudinal muscle usually retains its smooth appearance, while the inner, circular muscle which is cut through during the initial dissection assumes a fluffy appearance and tends to curve around the longitudinal muscle. To start the dissection, insert one closed pair of forceps between these two layers and then gently open and close them. The myenteric plexus generally adheres more to the circular muscle layer which is then removed as shown.

7. Transfer freed segments to cold BSS, using a Pasteur pipette.

8. Remove the last adherent muscle/connective tissue—this can be seen as a very fine translucent film between the ganglia.

9. Transfer the ganglia for a further rinse in culture medium before explanting (see section 4.2) or dissociating (see *Protocol 6*).

Using *Protocol 2* it is possible to obtain some 20 segments of plexus per animal. The size of the segments can be varied by using short or long strips of taenia coli. Large segments of dissected plexus can be divided using a sharp pair of iridectomy scissors. An example of a fairly small segment is shown in *Figure 2*. Because of the irregular nature of the plexus in this part of the gut, it is not possible to count the precise number of ganglia or to estimate the numbers of neurons per segment.

If, during the initial dissection, the lumen is pierced so the segments of gut are exposed to intestinal contents, the tissue must be cleaned by washing in HBSS and gently removing adherent intestinal contents with watchmaker's forceps. After inspection under a dissecting microscope to ensure all visible contents have been removed, the tissue is then rinsed twice in HBSS containing the antibiotic gentamycin (200 µg/ml) and the antiprotozoan metronidazole (Flagyl, Flow, 50 µg/ml). (A double-strength solution can be stored at 4 °C.) The tissue is then processed as described in *Protocol 2*.

3.1.2 Myenteric ganglia from the guinea-pig ileum or colon or rat intestine

Myenteric ganglia from these areas are obtained from segments of the entire intestinal wall, typically from 7–21 day animals, by a modification of the method used for the guinea-pig taenia coli (see *Protocol 3*). Tissue must be treated with antibiotics before enzyme treatment (see section 3.1.1). Overnight storage of tissue at 4 °C is **not** recommended for these tissues. However, a short period of approximately 2 h at 4 °C to allow enzyme penetration before incubation at 37 °C for 30–60 min has been found to aid sub-

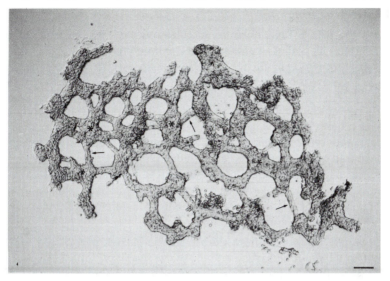

Figure 2. A small segment of the myenteric plexus dissected from beneath the taenia coli of a new-born guinea-pig. Myenteric ganglia (examples labelled with *) and interconnecting strands (examples labelled with *arrows*) can be seen. Scale bar represents 100 µm.

sequent dissection. Dissection of the plexus is also facilitated by use of good quality fine watchmaker's forceps, good illumination, and especially for rat plexus, high magnification ($\times$ 30–40). The isolated plexus segments should be transferred to cold BSS/medium before a final cleaning step with watch-maker's forceps at high magnification which is essential to remove all residual connective/muscular tissue which adheres to the plexus.

Protocol 3. Isolation of myenteric ganglia from guinea-pig or rat gut

Equipment and reagents
- As for *Protocol 2*

Method

1. Remove the intestine, place in BSS.
2. Trim off the mesentery.
3. Open the intestine along the side of mesenteric attachment.
4. Clean away the intestinal contents using forceps, and check micro-scopically that all contents have been removed.
5. Wash the tissue twice in antibiotic solution (see section 3.1.1).
6. Transfer to 1 mg/ml collagenase.

Protocol 3. *Continued*

7. Cut the tissue, parallel to the circular muscle, into pieces of about 2–3 mm in length (but of the entire circumference).

8. Place at 4 °C for 2 h.

9. Incubate at 37 °C for 30–50 min.

10. Using the dissecting microscope at x 30–40 magnification and fine watchmaker's forceps, separate strips of the outer longitudinal muscle, with adherent myenteric plexus. Illumination is crucial at this stage—it should be adjustable and arranged to illuminate the cut edge of the tissue so that the boundary between the longitudinal and circular muscle is easily discerned. Longitudinal muscle with plexus is best obtained using a gentle scraping/peeling movement, starting at a cut edge where the boundary is clearly visible.

11. Separate the muscle from the myenteric plexus, taking care not to pull at the nervous tissue.

12. Transfer the isolated ganglia to cold BSS/medium for final cleaning step.

The separation of the tissue layers described in *Protocol 3* should be easy to perform. If not, it is likely that the tissue has had an inappropriate incubation time in collagenase or, possibly, the batch of collagenase is suboptimal. It is recommended that an initial incubation of about 30 min is performed. If the tissue seems tough and hard to separate, it may be incubated for a further 10–20 min at 37 °C. If the enzyme solution becomes too acidic during incubation, it can be buffered with Hepes (e.g. 20 mM). The dissection may be quite lengthy, particularly for the beginner. If so, the tissue may become very soft/sloppy. To avoid this, transfer tissue to cold BSS, after about 1 h at room temperature.

3.2 Submucous plexus ganglia

Submucosal ganglia are dissected from the submucosa after enzyme treatment of pieces of the entire gut wall. Isolation of large numbers of submucous plexus ganglia by microdissection is difficult, since the ganglia are small and the interconnecting strands are relatively long and thin.

4. Explant cultures of isolated ganglia

The majority of studies of isolated enteric ganglia in culture have employed an explant culture technique.

4.1 Culture chambers, substrates, and media

Although isolated ganglia can be explanted into Petri dishes, modified Rose chambers have proved to be convenient culture chambers (13). These chambers consist of two glass coverslips separated by a gas permeable silicon gasket and are held together by metal clips. For subsequent ease of handling, segments can be explanted on to 13 mm glass coverslips (e.g. one explant/coverslip) which are then assembled into Rose chambers or placed in Petri dishes or multiwells. The coverslips may be uncoated or pre-coated with one (or more) of several substrates. When provided with serum-supplemented culture medium, enteric ganglia can be grown on plastic, glass, poly-L-lysine, collagen, laminin, or fibronectin substrates.

Enteric ganglion explant cultures have typically been grown either in serum-supplemented medium 199 or Dulbecco's modified Eagles medium. Culture media are usually supplemented with glucose (2–5 mg/ml), fetal calf serum (10%), and penicillin (100 U/ml). Streptomycin (100 µg/ml) and insulin (5 µg/ml) have also sometimes been included in the culture medium. However, it is likely that enteric ganglia can be grown successfully in a variety of other media. Serum-free, hormone-supplemented media have also been used for myenteric plexus cultures (see section 4.3.2).

4.2 Method of explantation

For explantation, each segment of plexus is transferred, using a Pasteur pipette, on to the culture substrate. After removal of excess medium from around the plexus with a fire-polished Pasteur, adherence of the plexus is further aided by drawing additional residual medium away from the explant with the ends of watchmaker forceps (care must be taken not to touch the tissue with the forceps, or to let the tissue dry out). The chamber is then closed and angled at 45–60° to the vertical for a few minutes before medium is introduced.

Submucous plexus ganglia are explanted in a similar manner to myenteric plexus ganglia, but subsequent growth is facilitated by covering the explants with a strip (1–2 mm wide) of sterile dialysis cellophane. This is conveniently achieved in a Rose chamber, where the cellophane can be sandwiched between the gasket and coverslip.

4.3 Guinea-pig myenteric plexus explants

4.3.1 Serum-supplemented medium

When grown in serum-supplemented medium, guinea-pig myenteric plexus explants undergo a characteristic pattern of growth in culture (6). The cultures contain enteric neurons and glial cells—any remaining adherent fibroblasts may be eliminated by the addition of cytosine arabinoside, at a concentration of $1–2 \times 10^{-5}$ M, for the first two to three days *in vitro*. The pattern of growth of these cultures over the first few days in culture is such that the organization of the plexus into linked ganglia is lost; enteric glial cells migrate from the ganglia to fill the holes of the network and form an outgrowth area over which enteric neurites regenerate. This process con-

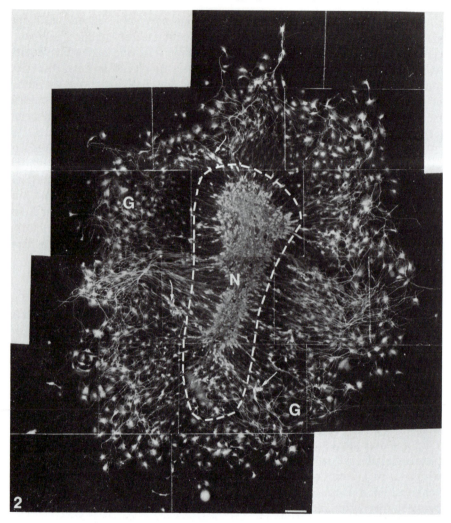

Figure 3. Immunofluorescence micrograph of a myenteric plexus explant culture grown in serum-supplemented medium, after five days *in vitro*, immunolabelled with an anti-serum to protein gene product 9.5. The majority of neuronal cell bodies, together with some glial cells, are confined to the central area (N). The surrounding outgrowth area (G) consists of enteric glial cells covered by regenerating enteric neurites. Occasional enteric neuronal cell bodies are present in this area of the cultures (examples indicated by *arrows*). The area which is excised in order to obtain enriched cultures of enteric glia (see *Protocol 5*) is indicated by the dashed lines. Scale bar represents 500 μm.

tinues over the next week to ten days. The enteric neuronal cell bodies, together with some enteric glial cells, are predominantly localized to the central area of the cultures, while an extensive outgrowth area consisting of enteric glial cells and overlying enteric neurites is formed peripherally

(*Figure 3*). At this time individual enteric neurons are clearly visible and accessible. In the absence of fibroblasts, this organization is maintained for the remainder of the culture period. However, if mitotic inhibitors are not employed, explants with many adherent fibroblasts undergo a different pattern of growth in which fibroblasts proliferate and the neural elements aggregate together into compact groups which show a number of similarities to enteric ganglia *in situ* (6,14).

4.3.2 Serum-free medium

Myenteric plexus explant cultures may also be grown in a serum-free medium (a modification of the N1 medium of Bottenstein *et al.*, 15; see ref. 16). In order to promote attachment of explants in the complete absence of serum, a laminin or fibronectin substrate may be used—enteric ganglion explants will not adhere in the absence of serum on glass or poly-L-lysine substrates (17). As with many other cell types, enteric glial cell migration and proliferation are reduced in serum-free culture (see ref. 18).

4.4 Rat myenteric plexus explants

Myenteric ganglia may be readily dissected from both ileum and colon of 7–21-day-old rats, and exhibit only a slightly different pattern of growth to those from the guinea-pig gut (6). Neuronal survival and neurite outgrowth are enhanced by growth in astrocyte conditioned medium (see Chapter 7).

4.5 Guinea-pig submucous plexus explants

Submucous plexus ganglia do not exhibit the same patterns of growth as myenteric plexus explants (6). Submucosal neurons tend to grow more successfully in explant culture when placed under a strip of dialysis cellophane, which may create a self-conditioning microenvironment.

5. Purified populations of enteric ganglion cells

The pattern of growth exhibited by myenteric plexus explants described above, together with the differential expression of some cell surface antigens by enteric neurons and glial cells, facilitates their use for the preparation of enriched cultures of neurons and glial cells (8).

5.1 Enteric neurons

Cultures enriched for myenteric neurons can be prepared from explant cultures of myenteric plexus by the combined use of mitotic inhibitors and complement killing (see *Protocol 4*). Cultures are explanted as described above, but are continuously exposed to cytosine arabinoside, which destroys not only fibroblasts but also many enteric glial cells. After 15–20 days in culture, remaining glial cells are almost completely eliminated by complement killing using a monoclonal antibody, LB1 (see ref. 19), which recognizes GD3 ganglioside expressed on the glial cell surfaces. After four to six weeks *in vitro*, such cultures typically contain between 78% and 96% neurons; remaining non-neuronal cells have been identified as fibroblasts (8).

Protocol 4. Preparation of enriched cultures of myenteric neurons

Equipment and reagents
- Equipment used for replacement of medium
- Culture medium
- Cytosine arabinoside
- LB1 antibody
- Rabbit complement

Method

1. Explant myenteric plexus segments as described in *Protocol 2*.
2. Provide with serum-supplemented medium containing 2×10^{-5} M cytosine arabinoside (medium is renewed twice weekly).
3. After 15–20 days in culture, incubate cultures in LB1 (ascites, diluted to 1 : 200, in medium) and complement (rabbit complement, 1 : 20) for 8 min at 37 °C.
4. After a further five days in culture, assess microscopically and either wash gently to remove dead glial cells and then replace medium, or re-treat with LB1 and complement. Two treatments with LB1 and complement are generally required in order to remove all glia.

5.2 Enteric glial cells

Cultures enriched for enteric glial cells can be prepared from myenteric plexus explants using a combination of three methods; treatment with mitotic inhibitors to remove fibroblasts, excision of the central neuronal area after seven days *in vitro*, and complement killing to remove residual neurons and fibroblasts (see *Protocol 5*). Using this approach, cultures containing more than 98% enteric glial cells can be obtained, after 17 days *in vitro* (8).

Protocol 5. Preparation of enriched cultures of myenteric glial cells

Equipment and reagents
- Equipment used for replacement of medium
- Culture medium
- Cytosine arabinoside
- Sterile 21 gauge needle
- Dissecting microscope
- Anti-Thy-1 antibody (e.g. ref. 20)
- Rabbit complement
- Sterile Pasteur pipette

Method

1. Explant myenteric plexus segments as described in *Protocol 2*.

2. Provide with serum-supplemented medium containing 2 x 10^{-5} M cytosine arabinoside for the first six days in culture.

3. After seven days in culture, excise the central neuronal area using the bent end of a sterile 21 gauge needle, under a dissecting microscope at x 20–40 magnification (see *Figure 3*). Discard excised cells using a Pasteur pipette.

4. Treat remaining cells with Thy-1 antibody (1 : 100) and complement (1 : 20) for 45–60 min at 37 °C.

5. Return coverslips to medium, continue to feed twice weekly. A second complement killing can be performed if necessary.

Such enriched cultures have been used to examine the effects of various agents on the proliferation of enteric glial cells (see ref. 4). However, they have the disadvantage that the purified populations of cells are only obtained after a considerable time in culture.

6. Dissociated cell cultures of postnatal enteric ganglion cells

Several different methods for the preparation of dissociated cell cultures of enteric neurons have been published (see section 2). However, apart from dissociates obtained from enteric ganglia which have previously been separated from the gut wall by dissection, enteric neurons are heavily outnumbered by non-neuronal cells in these preparations.

6.1 Dissociation of isolated enteric ganglia

Segments of myenteric plexus dissected from the guinea-pig or rat gut can be dissociated to give a cell suspension consisting of enteric neurons and glial cells (7). Further manipulation of such suspensions may permit purified populations of neurons or glia to be obtained.

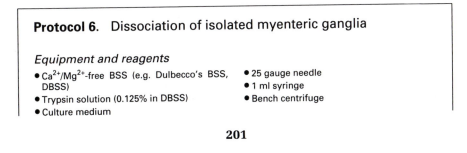

Protocol 6. Dissociation of isolated myenteric ganglia

Equipment and reagents
- Ca^{2+}/Mg^{2+}-free BSS (e.g. Dulbecco's BSS, DBSS)
- Trypsin solution (0.125% in DBSS)
- Culture medium
- 25 gauge needle
- 1 ml syringe
- Bench centrifuge

Protocol 6. *Continued*

Method

1. Isolate segments of myenteric plexus by microdissection as in *Protocol 2* or *3*. To obtain large numbers of cells it is necessary to use tissue from several animals.

2. Rinse segments in Ca^{2+}/Mg^{2+}-free BSS.

3. Transfer to 0.125% trypsin in BSS.

4. Incubate at 4°C for 2 h.

5. Incubate at 37°C for 30 min.

6. Spin gently.

7. Tip off trypsin solution, add culture medium.

8. Pass through 25 gauge needle on 1 ml syringe, four to six times.

Using this method to dissociate myenteric ganglia from the guinea-pig taenia coli, it is possible to obtain some 7×10^5 enteric ganglion cells from four animals. The cell suspension contains both enteric neurons and glia. The yield of cells and their dispersal may be aided by the inclusion of DNase in the incubation media. In order to obtain enriched populations of neurons or glia, techniques such as pre-plating, complement killing or immunoselection, and/or the use of mitotic inhibitors is necessary. To date, these methods have not been widely applied to enteric ganglion cell cultures from isolated ganglia.

Recently, another method for obtaining increased amounts of myenteric plexus from the rat gut has been reported. The method involves a combination of collagenase and mechanical treatment of the muscularis externa, after which freed plexus segments are harvested with the aid of a dissecting microscope. (See Schäfer K.-H., Saffrey, M. J., and Burnstock, G. (1995). *Neuroreport*, **6,** 937.)

Acknowledgements

This work has been supported by the Medical Research Council of Great Britain and the Wellcome Trust.

References

1. Furness, J. B. and Costa, M. (1987). *The enteric nervous system*. Churchill-Livingstone, Edinburgh.
2. Gabella, G. (1979). *Int. Rev. Cytol.*, **59,** 129.

3. Jessen, K. R. and Burnstock, G. (1982). In *Trends in autonomic pharmacology* (ed. S. Kalsner), pp. 95–115. Urban and Schwarzenberg, Baltimore.
4. Saffrey, M. J., Hassall, C. J. S., Allen, T. G. J., and Burnstock, G. (1992). *Int. Rev. Cytol.*, **136,** 93.
5. Jessen, K. R., McConnell, J. D., Purves, R. D., Burnstock, G., and Chamley-Campbell, J. (1978). *Brain Res.*, **152,** 573.
6. Jessen, K. R., Saffrey, M. J., and Burnstock, G. (1983). *Brain Res.*, **262,** 17.
7. Saffrey, M. J., Bailey, D. J., and Burnstock, G. (1991). *Cell Tissue Res.*, **265,** 527.
8. Bannerman, P. G. C., Mirsky, R., and Jessen, K. R. (1988). *Brain Res.*, **440,** 99.
9. Nishi, R. and Willard, A. L. (1985). *Neuroscience*, **16,** 187.
10. Willard, A. L. and Nishi, R. (1989). In *Handbook of physiology* (ed. S. G. Shultz, J. D. Wood, and B. B. Rauner), Section 6, Vol. 1, pp. 331–47. Oxford University Press, New York.
11. Barber, D. L., Buchan, A. M. J., Leeman, S. E., and Soll, A. H. (1989). *Neuroscience*, **32,** 145.
12. Pomeranz, H. D., Rothman, T. P., Chalazonitis, A., Tennyson, V. M., and Gershon, M. D. (1993). *Dev. Biol.*, **156,** 341.
13. Rose, G. (1954). *Tex. Rep. Biol. Med.*, **12,** 1074.
14. Baluk, P., Jessen, K. R., Saffrey, M. J., and Burnstock, G. (1983). *Brain Res.*, **262,** 37.
15. Bottenstein, J. E., Skaper, S. D., Varon, S. S., and Sato, G. (1980). *Exp. Cell Res.*, **125,** 183.
16. Saffrey, M. J. and Burnstock, G. (1984). *Intl. J. Dev. Neurosci.*, **2,** 591.
17. Saffrey, M. J. and Burnstock, G. (1992). *Intl. J. Dev. Neurosci.*, **10,** 97.
18. Eccleston, P. A., Bannerman, P. G. C., Pleasure, D. E., Winter, J., Mirsky, R., and Jessen, K. R. (1989). *Development*, **107,** 107.
19. Levi, G., Gallo, V., Wilkin, G. P., and Cohen, J. (1986). In *Advances in the biosciences* (ed. T. Grisar), Vol. 61, pp. 21–30. Pergamon, Oxford.
20. Williams, A. F. and Gagnon, J. (1982). *Science*, **216,** 696.

Mouse olfactory epithelium

ANNE L. CALOF, JOSE L. GUEVARA, and
MELINDA K. GORDON

1. Introduction

The olfactory epithelium is unique in mammals in that proliferation of neuronal precursor cells and differentiation of their progeny into olfactory receptor neurons (ORNs) continue throughout the lifetime of the organism (1,2). Many of the studies in our laboratory are concerned with understanding how specific polypeptide growth factors and cell interactions regulate olfactory receptor neuron generation and survival (3–6). For these studies it is crucial to obtain and culture explants of olfactory epithelium that are free from stromal cells, since the stromal cells may provide signals that affect the development of olfactory receptor neurons. Thus, an entire section of this chapter is devoted to purification of the epithelium from its underlying stroma. For studies of growth factor effects on isolated ORNs, and for studies on olfactory receptor neuron adhesion, migration, and axon outgrowth, we prepare a neuronal cell fraction from embryonic mouse olfactory epithelium, as well as using explant cultures. This neuronal cell fraction consists solely of olfactory receptor neurons and their precursors, which we have called the immediate neuronal precursors (INPs) of olfactory receptor neurons, and does not contain basal cells or supporting (sustentacular) cells of the epithelium (6–8). Using this cell fraction allows us to work solely with neuronal cells in dissociated cell culture, which is a great advantage for quantitative studies.

Other authors have published methods for culturing olfactory epithelium from both embryonic and neonatal rats, and the reader is referred to these papers for culture methods for rat tissue (e.g. 9–17). However, because of the availability of many strains of transgenic mice that are of interest for studies on olfactory neurogenesis and development (6,18–22), as well as the greater ease of maintaining mouse as opposed to rat breeding colonies, the mouse is the preferred species for our studies.

2. Dissection and purification of olfactory epithelium from mouse embryos

We perform all the procedures described below on the bench-top in a room used exclusively for dissection. In order to maintain sterility, we wipe down all surfaces with 70% ethanol before beginning a preparation, and routinely dip our instruments in 95% ethanol and flame them. All procedures are performed using sterile, disposable polystyrene dishes and either sterile polystyrene tissue culture pipettes or autoclaved 9 inch Pasteur pipettes.

In order to work with precisely timed embryos, it is usually necessary to maintain your own breeding colony. For most of our experiments, we use random-bred CD-1 (Swiss) mice from Charles River Laboratories. The mice are naturally mated, and females are checked every morning for the presence of a vaginal plug, which indicates successful mating. The date of the vaginal plug is designated day 0.5 of pregnancy. For explant cultures, embryos are taken at day 14.5 or 15.5 of pregnancy. For dissociated cell culture, we purify epithelium from embryos taken any time from day 14.5 to day 17.5 of pregnancy, depending upon the goal of the particular experiment.

2.1 Dissection

Preparation of the olfactory epithelium (OE) for culture involves first, dissection of turbinates from the nasal cavities, and secondly, purification of the OE itself from its underlying stroma, which consists primarily of fibroblasts and chondrocytes. The dissection procedure has three parts:

- removal of the embryos from the pregnant mouse (see Barker and Johnson, Chapter 3 for procedure)
- dissection of heads into hemi-snouts
- removal of olfactory turbinates from the hemi-snouts

Once the embryos have been removed from the pregnant mouse, all subsequent procedures are performed using a dissection microscope equipped with bright-field and dark-field transillumination. Fibre-optic illumination is useful in the initial removal of turbinates from hemi-snouts.

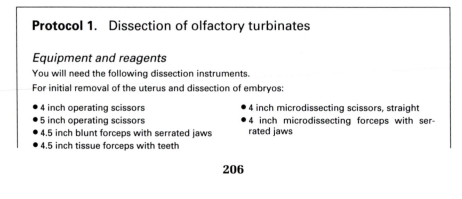

Protocol 1. Dissection of olfactory turbinates

Equipment and reagents

You will need the following dissection instruments.

For initial removal of the uterus and dissection of embryos:

- 4 inch operating scissors
- 5 inch operating scissors
- 4.5 inch blunt forceps with serrated jaws
- 4.5 inch tissue forceps with teeth
- 4 inch microdissecting scissors, straight
- 4 inch microdissecting forceps with serrated jaws

For removal of the olfactory turbinates from embryo heads:

- Tissue culture PBS with serum (for dissection of heads and removal of turbinates): to 500 ml of cold 1 x PBS (prepared as described in Appendix), add 25 ml bovine calf serum, defined, iron supplemented (Hyclone, A2151L, or equivalent high quality, virus and endotoxin-free bovine calf serum), and 2.5 ml penicillin–streptomycin, 10000 U/ml (Gibco-BRL, 15140–015), store at 4°C

- Dumont No. 5 microdissecting forceps
- 3.5 inch Castroviejo ultra microscissors, angular, blades 11 mm, sharp ends (Roboz, RS-5658)[a]

Method

1. After removing the embryos from the pregnant mouse, decapitate the embryos and place the heads on ice in a 100 mm Petri dish containing cold PBS with serum. Distribute the heads into 60 mm Petri dishes, with three or four heads in each dish. Make the first, coronal incision from the top to the base of the head, and remove the entire back of the head (see *Figure 1A*). Do this for all the heads in the dish. Remove the waste tissue (backs of heads) from the dissection dish.

2. Place each head standing up on the surface that was just cut, and make the second, horizontal incision to remove the lower jaw and tongue (*Figure 1B*). Remove this waste tissue from the dissection dish. Make the third, sagittal incision from the front of the snout through the back of the head, splitting the front part of the head and the nasal cavity into two halves ('hemi-snouts').

3. Lay the two hemi-snouts on their sides, so that the inside of the nasal cavity is face up. The olfactory turbinates (O.T.) appear as oval buds covered by a shiny, translucent layer of cells (the olfactory epithelium) (*Figure 1C*). The invaginations in the surface of the turbinates appear as dark lines running crosswise across the ovals. In about half of the hemi-snouts, the turbinate will not be visible because it is covered by the nasal septum (N.S.). If the septum is peeled away with fine forceps, then the turbinate should be visible. Place the tips of the fine forceps underneath each turbinate, and pinch gently to remove it (*Figure 1D*).

[a] While most of the instruments are readily available from a number of different sources, we have found that the Castroviejo ultra microdissecting scissors from Roboz (or Downs Surgical, see Appendix) work particularly well for the incisions of the embryo heads.

Protocol 2. Purification of OE

Reagents

- Holding medium for turbinates: 575 ml of cold 1 x PBS, 0.6 ml phenol red, 0.5% (Gibco-BRL, 630–5100AG), 3 ml penicillin–streptomycin (10000 U/ml), 6 ml 30% glucose, dissolved in H_2O, 25 ml fetal bovine serum (Hyclone, A-1111-L)—filter sterilize with 0.2 μm filter, and store at 4 °C
- Post-trypsin rinse: 500 ml cold 1 x PBS, 5 ml 30% glucose, 0.5 ml phenol red, 0.5%, 2.5 ml penicillin–streptomycin (10000 U/ml), 250 mg albumin, bovine, crystalline (BSA; ICN Biomedicals, 103700), 125 mg trypsin inhibitor, Type I-S from soybean (Sigma, T-9003)—sterilize through 0.2 μm filter, and store at 4 °C
- Trituration medium: 500 ml cold 1 x PBS, 5 ml 30% glucose, 2.5 ml penicillin–streptomycin (10000 U/ml), 0.5 ml phenol red, 0.5%, 250 mg crystalline BSA (ICN Biomedicals, 103700)—sterilize though 0.2 μm filter, and store at 4 °C

- Trypsin–pancreatin solution (for separation of olfactory epithelium from stroma): in a 250 ml polypropylene centrifuge bottle add 1 g pancreatin, from porcine pancreas, Grade II (Sigma, P-1500), 3 g trypsin 1 : 250 (Difco Laboratories, Detroit, MI), 0.5 ml phenol red, 0.5%, 1 ml penicillin–streptomycin (10000 U/ml), 100 ml cold 1 x PBS. Mix well to dissolve, keeping at 4 °C. Spin 20 min at ~ 16300 *g* to remove insoluble material. Filter supernatant twice through Whatman No. 1 filter paper, keeping solution on ice. Filter sterilize through 0.2 μm filter unit with pre-filter. Make 8 ml aliquots and store in sterile polypropylene tubes at −20 °C.

Method

1. As you dissect the turbinates out of the heads in each dish, collect the turbinates by mouth pipette, using a sterile, cotton plugged 9 inch Pasteur pipette attached to a plastic mouthpiece with latex tubing (*Figure 1E*). Transfer the turbinates to a separate 60 mm Petri dish, on ice, containing holding medium. Collect all the turbinates from a dissection into this dish, then remove the holding medium using a sterile Pasteur pipette (being careful not to lose any turbinates), rinse the turbinates once in ice-cold PBS, remove the PBS, and add 8 ml of trypsin–pancreatin solution.

2. Incubate the turbinates in the trypsin–pancreatin solution for 40–55 min on ice, depending on the age of the embryos (40 min for E14.5, 50–55 min for E16.5–17.5). Then remove the enzyme solution and add 8–10 ml of post-trypsin rinse to the dish. Keep dish on ice.

3. Transfer the turbinates into 35 mm Petri dishes each containing 2.5 ml of cold trituration medium (*Figure 1F*). Distribute two turbinates into each dish, again by mouth pipette.

4. To remove the OE from its underlying stroma, gently triturate the turbinates using a hand-held 9 inch Pasteur pipette whose opening has been flamed down to approximately the width of the turbinates (*Figire 1F, 1*). Under dark-field illumination, draw the turbinates up and down in the pipette, and the epithelium will separate from the stroma (*Figure 1F, 2*). The epithelium may still have some stroma

attached (*Figure 1F*, 3), however, so it is necessary to continue triturating until there is no stroma attached to the epithelium (*Figure 1F*, 4).
The epithelium will appear as shiny, translucent sheets in dark-field
transillumination, whereas the stroma will appear as irregularly
shaped, opaque masses of cells and collagen fibrils.

5. Transfer purified pieces of epithelium by mouth pipette through two
   successive rinses of low calcium culture medium (see *Protocol 4*),
   each in a new 60 mm Petri dish held on ice. Inspect each piece of
   epithelium during the first rinse, and carefully remove any remaining
   stroma before transferring the epithelium to the second, medium-con-
   taining dish.

3. Culturing olfactory epithelium explants

In our explant culture system, small pieces of OE are plated on to substrata
that maximize neuronal migration. Three cell types are readily identifiable
within one day of initiating olfactory epithelium explant cultures:

(a) Basal cells remain within the body of the explant, and grow as sheets of
epithelial cells that express keratins (3,4).

(b) Immature olfactory receptor neurons migrate readily from explants that
have been cultured on merosin- or laminin-treated substrata (3,7,8). The
immature olfactory receptor neurons are postmitotic cells that can be
easily recognized in culture by their neurites; in addition, they are the
only cells in the OE that express the neural cell adhesion molecule
NCAM, which can be recognized by several different antibodies (3–5,7).

(c) The immediate neuronal precursors (INPs) of olfactory receptor neurons
are also present in these cultures within the first 24–48 h (3–6). INPs do
not express keratins or NCAM, and they can be recognized as migratory,
round cells that rapidly sort out from the body of the explant, synthesizing DNA and dividing as they migrate. [^{3}H]Thymidine incorporation
analysis has shown that the INPs are the direct precursors of olfactory
receptor neurons (3–5). Thus, the disappearance of NCAM-negative
INPs from olfactory epithelium cultures is a result of these cells giving
rise to postmitotic olfactory receptor neurons, which express NCAM.

In addition to the three major cell types described above, our recent studies—
using an antibody to a mucin expressed by sustentacular cells of the olfactory
epithelium (23)—suggest that sustentacular cells and basal cells may be inter-
mixed within some of the epithelial sheets that develop in embryonic olfactory
epithelium cultures (24) (A. Calof and S. Whitehead, unpublished results).
We have also shown that olfactory Schwann cells (ensheathing cells) may

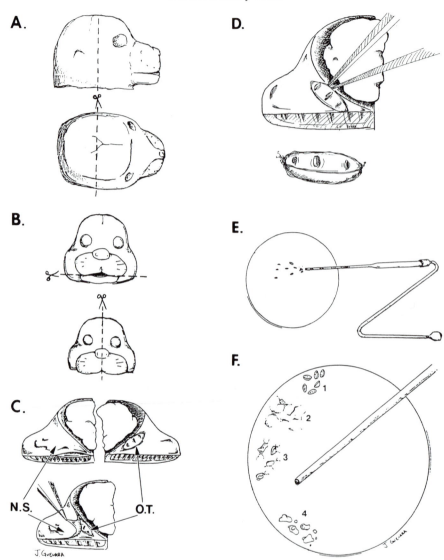

Figure 1. Dissection of olfactory turbinates and purification of olfactory epithelium. See *Protocols 1* and *2*.

appear in long-term OE cultures (24). For immunocytochemical procedures see section 5.

3.1   Preparation of substrata for explant cultures

For explant culture of OE, we use acid-cleaned glass coverslips that have been coated with one of several extracellular matrix molecules. For olfactory receptor neuron axon outgrowth and cell migration, laminin or its homologue merosin are the best substrata; however, fibronectin is an excellent substratum for epithelial attachment (3,7). We have found the best 'compromise' is to coat coverslips with poly-D-lysine (Sigma, P-0899, 1 mg/ml in ddH$_2$O, 4 h to overnight), then wash them four times with ddH$_2$O, and sterilize by ultraviolet irradiation. The coverslips are then coated with merosin (Gibco-BRL, 12162–012) at 10 µg/ml in Ca^{2+}/Mg^{2+}-free Hank's balanced salt solution (CMF-HBSS; Cellgro Mediatech, 21–021-LM) for 3 h at 37 °C. After rinsing four times in sterile CMF-HBSS, the coverslips are placed into the wells of a 24-well tissue culture tray (we use Falcon, 3047), covered in low calcium culture medium, and explants are plated on to them.

Protocol 3.   Acid cleaning glass coverslips for tissue culture

1. Place one ounce of round glass coverslips (12 mm, No. 1 thinness; Propper Manufacturing, Long Island City, NY) into 500 ml of 1% HCl in ddH$_2$O in a 2 litre Pyrex beaker.

2. In a fume hood, boil the coverslips in the HCl solution for 1–3 h, stirring frequently with a glass rod.

3. Pour off the HCl solution, and add 500 ml ddH$_2$O to the beaker. Bring the water to the boil, and then pour off. Do this three times.

4. After the third rinse in boiling ddH$_2$O, rinse the coverslips once in 95% ethanol, swirling gently.

5. Discard the ethanol, cover the beaker loosely with aluminium foil, and dry the coverslips in a vacuum oven set at 60 °C overnight.

3.2   Culture media

All of our tissue culture media are made with a lower level of calcium than is present in most tissue culture media (0.1 mM as opposed to 2 mM), since we have found this to be optimal for cell sorting and cell migration in cultures of mouse OE (3,7). The basal medium used for culturing OE consists of two-thirds calcium-free DME (see *Protocol 4*), and one-third Ham's F-12; this medium is supplemented with additives to promote cell growth.

3.3 Culturing explants

In many of our studies, we analyse the effects of pharmacological agents and polypeptide growth factors on purified olfactory epithelium grown on the substrata described above. Chopping the OE into small pieces increases the number of explants which can be analysed.

Protocol 4. Low calcium OE culture medium

Reagents

- Calcium-free DME: to a 500 ml tissue culture bottle (preferably a new polystyrene bottle) add 50 ml 10 x Earle's balanced salt solution with phenol red (Ca^{2+}/Mg^{2+}-free; Gibco-BRL, 14160–022), 5.833 ml 30% glucose, 5 ml 100 x $MgSO_4 \cdot 7H_2O$ (20 mg/ml in ddH_2O), 10 ml MEM amino acids solution without L-glutamine, 50 x(Gibco-BRL, 11130–010), 5 ml MEM non-essential amino acids, 10 mM, 100 x (Gibco-BRL, 320–1140AG), 5 ml MEM vitamins solution, 100 x (Gibco-BRL, 11120–11), 0.5 ml phenol red 0.5%, 0.5 ml 1000 x $Fe(NO_3) \cdot 9H_2O$ (10 mg/litre in ddH_2O), 1.1 g $NaHCO_3$, take up to final volume of 500 ml with ddH_2O—filter through 0.2 µm filter to sterilize, and store at 4 °C

- Serum-free additives (100 x stock): to 60 ml Ca^{2+}/Mg^{2+}-free Hank's balanced salt solution (CMF-HBSS; Cellgro Mediatech, 21–021-LM) add 10 ml insulin (Sigma, I 5500), 10 mg/ml in 10 mM HCl, 100 mg transferrin (Sigma, T 1283), 100 µl progesterone (Sigma, P 8783), 2 mM in 100% ethanol, 10 ml putrescine (Sigma, P 5780), 100 mM (16.11 mg/ml) in CMF-HBSS, 100 µl sodium selenite (Sigma, S 5261), 3 mM (519 µg/ml) in CMF-HBSS, 200 mg crystalline BSA, take to a final volume of 100 ml with CMF-HBSS—filter sterilize (0.2 µm), make 1–2 ml aliquots in sterile polypropylene tubes, and store at –80 °C

Serum-free additives are a modification of the additives devised by Bottenstein and Sato for the growth of neuroblastoma cells (25). The final concentration of the additives in the culture medium is: insulin, 10 µg/ml; transferrin, 10 µg/ml; progesterone, 20 nM; putrescine, 100 µM; and selenium, 30 nM.

Method

1. To prepare the medium, first add 500 mg crystalline BSA to 70 ml calcium-free DME, and mix until the BSA has dissolved. The resulting solution will be acidic (the medium will be yellow), and should be neutralized by adding 1 M NaOH dropwise (50–100 µl is usually sufficient to the restore the pH, turning the medium pink again).

2. Add the following:
   - 35 ml Ham's F-12 with L-glutamine (Cellgro Mediatech, 10–080-LV)
   - 0.5 ml penicillin–streptomycin (10 000 U/ml)
   - 1 ml L-glutamine, 200 mM, 100 x (Gibco-BRL, 320–5030AG)
   - 1.15 ml serum-free additives, 100 x

3. Sterilize by filtering through a 0.2 µm filter.

4. Store at 4 °C.

Protocol 5. Explant culture

1. After transferring the isolated epithelium to the second dish of low calcium medium (*Protocol 2*), chop the OE into fine pieces using a sharp blade or knife (we use tungsten wire etched in 10% KOH).

2. After chopping, gently swirl the dish until all of the tissue is in the centre of the dish. Using a sterile Pasteur pipette, gently take up the pieces of epithelium, and distribute by mouth pipette on to acid-cleaned, treated coverslips which have been placed into the wells of a 24-well tissue culture tray and covered with low calcium medium (1.5 ml/well). Optimal density is obtained by using one 12 mm round coverslip for every three or four embryos dissected.

3. Incubate at 37 °C in a 5% CO_2 atmosphere.

3.4 Growth factor requirements

Explants prepared and cultured as described above will survive for several days. However, the INPs cease to divide unless they receive appropriate growth factor stimulation (5), and olfactory receptor neurons begin to die within this period unless they are grown in agents that inhibit programmed cell death (6,18,21). For example, aurintricarboxylic acid (100 µM; Sigma, A 0885) promotes the survival of dissociated olfactory receptor neurons (see section 4) at late times in culture (see *Figure 2C*). Basal cells of the epithelium require epidermal growth factor for their continued proliferation and survival (3,4). Ongoing studies in our laboratory are directed toward identifying specific polypeptide growth factors that will stimulate proliferation of INPs and promote long-term survival of olfactory receptor neurons. To date, we have found that members of the fibroblast growth factor family stimulate proliferation by INPs in explant cultures (5,18), and that individual members of the neurotrophin family will promote survival of small numbers of dissociated olfactory receptor neurons (see section 4), although no single neurotrophin will allow survival of all olfactory receptor neurons in a culture (6,18,21).

4. Culture of isolated neurons and neuronal precursors

In many of our experiments, we isolate the olfactory receptor neurons and their precursors (the immediate neuronal precursors, or INPs) from the basal cells of the epithelium. Immunocytochemical analysis has demonstrated that the cells in this fraction, referred to as the neuronal cell fraction, are either olfactory receptor neurons (~ 74%) or INPs (~ 26%) (5–7). Culturing these cells in the absence of the other OE cell types (i.e. basal cells and sustentacular cells) allows us to study directly the effects of growth factors and pharmacological agents on the neuronal population.

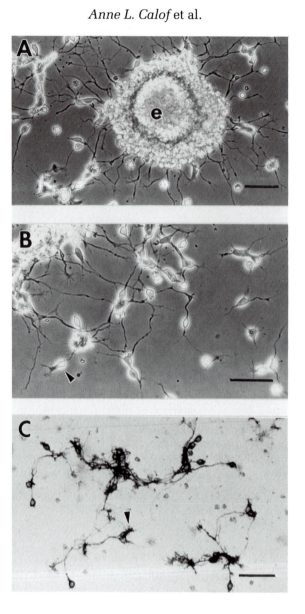

4.1 Preparation of substrata for dissociated neuronal cell fraction

Cultures of the dissociated neuronal cell fraction grow well at high density on tissue culture plastic coated with poly-D-lysine. For these studies, we coat the wells of 96-well tissue cultue trays (Costar, 3596) overnight at 4 °C with 50 µl/well of poly-D-lysine (1 mg/ml in ddH$_2$O). The plates are then washed five times in ddH$_2$O and sterilized by ultraviolet irradiation.

Figure 2. Olfactory epithelium and olfactory receptor neurons in explant and dissociated cell culture. (A) Explant of olfactory epithelium purified from E14 CD-1 mouse embryos and grown for 18 h in low calcium culture medium. The substratum is an acid-washed glass coverslip, coated with merosin. Note the many axonal processes and olfactory receptor neuron cell bodies that have migrated out of the epithelial explant ('e'), even at this early time in culture. Bar = 50 μm. (B) Higher power view of olfactory receptor neurons that have migrated out of an olfactory epithelium explant grown in the same conditions as in (A). The *arrowhead* points to an olfactory receptor neuron with a prominent dendrite. Bar = 50 μm. (C) Olfactory receptor neurons grown in dissociated cell culture in a polylysine coated 96-well tissue culture tray. After being cultured for 72 h in low calcium medium containing 100 μM aurintricarboxylic acid (6,18), the cells were fixed in Omnifix II and processed *in situ* for NCAM expression as described in section 5.1(b), using the Vector ABC-AP kit followed by a blue chromagen (Vector SK-5300 blue). Note the thick apical dendrites (*arrowhead*) and the thin axonal processes of the neurons. Bar = 50 μm.

4.2 Suspension culture and isolation of the neuronal cell fraction

The initial preparation of the neuronal cell fraction is identical to that of the olfactory epithelium explants. After isolating the purified epithelium, however, three new steps are added:

(a) The isolated epithelium is cultured in suspension for 6–12 h (during this time, olfactory receptor neurons and their precursors sort out from, but remain loosely attached to, the basal epithelial cells, which form a ball of tightly packed cells).

(b) The neuronal cell fraction is isolated from the basal cells by sequential enzymatic digestion and mechanical dissociation.

(c) Cells in the neuronal cell fraction are plated into the wells of tissue culture trays.

Protocol 6. Dissociation and isolation of olfactory neurons and neuronal precursors from suspension cultures

Equipment and reagents

The solutions should be sterilized by filtering with a 0.2 μm filter and stored at –20°C in 1–2 ml aliquots.

- Nylon mesh, 10 μm (CMN-10-D; Small Parts, Inc., Miami, FL)
- Trypsin solution (5 mg/ml): dissolve 100 mg trypsin (Sigma, T-8253) in 20 ml Leibovitz's L-15 medium (Gibco, 320–1415AJ)
- Trypsin inhibitor solution (5 mg/ml): dissolve 250 mg trypsin inhibitor (Type I-S from soybean; Sigma, T-9003) in 50 ml L-15
- Deoxyribonuclease (DNase) solution (1 mg/ml): dissolve 100 mg DNase I (Sigma, D-5025) in 100 ml Dulbecco's modification of Eagles medium (DME; Mediatech, 15-013-LV)
- 4% crystalline BSA: dissolve 4 g crystalline BSA in 100 ml CMF-HBSS

215

Protocol 6. *Continued*

Method

1. After collecting purified epithelium in the second dish of low calcium medium (see *Protocol 2*), transfer the epithelium to a third 60 mm Petri dish containing 8–10 ml low calcium medium. Incubate the cells in this dish for 6–12 h at 37 °C in a 5% CO_2 atmosphere.
2. Transfer the tissue from the suspension culture into a sterile 15 ml conical polystyrene centrifuge tube.
3. Rinse the suspension culture dish with 4–5 ml CMF-HBSS, and add the rinse to the centrifuge tube.
4. Spin for 5 min at 100 *g*.
5. After carefully aspirating the supernatant, add 4 ml CMF-HBSS to the tissue pellet.
6. Add 0.4 ml trypsin (5 mg/ml), and incubate in a 37 °C water-bath for 4 min.[a]
7. Add 1 ml of 1 mg/ml DNase to the cell suspension, swirl to mix, and return to the water-bath for 6 min.
8. Add 1 ml of 5 mg/ml trypsin inhibitor.
9. Mechanically dissociate the cells by triturating ten times using a flame-polished Pasteur pipette.
10. Let sit for 3 min (this allows the larger clumps, composed primarily of basal cells, to settle to the bottom of the tube).
11. Remove 4.5–5 ml from the top of the cell suspension, and filter this through sterile (autoclaved) 10 µm nylon mesh into another 15 ml conical centrifuge tube.
12. To the remaining cell suspension (approx. 1.5–2 ml) add 4 ml CMF-HBSS and 1 ml of 5 mg/ml trypsin inhibitor.
13. Repeat the trituration, settling, and filtration steps (9–11), collecting both filtrates in the same 15 ml conical centrifuge tube.
14. Underlay the filtered cell suspension with 2 ml 4% crystalline BSA (in CMF-HBSS), and spin for 10 min at 100 *g*.
15. Remove the supernatant by aspirating with a flame-polished Pasteur pipette, and resuspend the pellet in a small volume (~ 1.5 ml) of low calcium medium.
16. Use a haemocytometer to count the cells, and plate cells at the desired density into polylysine coated 96-well tissue culture trays (see section 4.1). For high density cultures, we typically plate ~ 3 x 10^4 cells/well of a 96-well tray.

[a] Alternatively, the trypsin may be replaced with 200 µl of 1 mg/ml dispase (Grade I, > 6 U/mg, made in L-15; Boehringer Mannheim, 210455), and incubated for 10 min at 37 °C; or the dissociation may be done without the use of proteolytic enzymes, by eliminating step 6 and proceeding directly to step 7 (eliminate all 37 °C incubations if no enzymes are used).

5. Analysis of cell types within olfactory epithelium cultures

Cell type specific markers have proved invaluable for analysing the generation, differentiation, and maturation of mouse olfactory receptor neurons, both *in vivo* and *in vitro* (3–6,18,21,22). Immunocytochemical analysis of the cell types present in mouse olfactory epithelium cultures can be performed using a number of different antibodies. We list below those antibodies that have been used successfully in our laboratory, along with the fixation conditions, and immunocytochemical procedures that we currently use.

5.1 Olfactory receptor neuron markers

(a) H28 anti-NCAM (neural cell adhesion molecule) (rat hybridoma): H28 rat IgG (kind gift of Christo Goridis) recognizes an extracellular domain common to all three forms of the NCAM polypeptide, and is used as full strength tissue culture supernatant (26) (also available from AMAC, Inc., Westbrook, ME; Cat. No. 0270). Fixation: 3.7% formaldehyde in PBS, 10 min at room temperature. Visualize with Texas red goat anti-rat IgG (Jackson), 1 : 50 dilution.

(b) AG1D5 anti-NCAM: mouse anti-NCAM ascites fluid diluted 1 : 500, or full strength tissue culture supernatant (3); recognizes a cytoplasmic domain common to the 140 and 180 kDa forms of NCAM. Fixation: acetone, room temperature, 5 min; or Omnifix II (An-Con Genetics, Inc., Melville, NY), 10 min. Visualize with rhodamine goat anti-mouse IgG (Tago), 1 : 100 dilution. This antibody can also be visualized with goat anti-mouse IgG biotin (Vector, 2.5 µg/ml), followed by alkaline phosphatase conjugated to avidin (Vector, AK-5000; alkaline phosphatase ABC kit).

(c) Anti-GAP43: sheep antiserum to GAP-43 (generous gift of L. Benowitz) used at a 1 : 1000 dilution (3) (a monoclonal anti-GAP-43 also available from Boehringer Mannheim, 1379 011). Fixation: 3.7% formaldehyde in PBS, 10 min at room temperature; permeablize with 0.1–0.2% Triton X-100 in PBS. Visualize with rabbit anti-sheep biotin (Vector; 2.5 µg/ml) followed by avidin–alkaline phosphatase (as specified in Vectastain ABC-AP kit).

5.2 Olfactory Schwann cell (ensheathing cell) markers

(a) Anti-S100: rabbit anti-S100 (Dako, Z311) use at a 1 : 200 dilution (24,27). Fixation: PPG (4% paraformaldehyde/0.2% picric acid/0.05 % glutaraldehyde/0.1 M sodium phosphate, pH 7.0), 15 min. Permeablize with 0.1–0.2% Triton X-100 in PBS. Visualize with FITC-conjugated goat anti-rabbit IgG (Capell), 1 : 100 dilution.

(b) Anti-GFAP (glial fibrillary acidic protein): rabbit anti-GFAP IgG (Dako, Z334) is used at 1 : 100 (24,27,28). Fixation: acetone. Visualize with FITC-conjugated goat anti-rabbit IgG (Capell), 1 : 100 dilution.

5.3 Sustentacular cell marker

3C2 anti-mucin: mouse hybridoma producing anti-mucin IgM (kind gift of Pat Levitt and Steve Prouty). Full strength hybridoma supernatant (23). Fixation: PPG, acetone, or Omnifix II. Visualize with Texas red goat anti-mouse IgM (Jackson), 1 : 100 dilution.

5.4 Basal cell marker

Anti-cytokeratin: Dako rabbit polyclonal anti-keratin (wide spectrum screening; Dakopatts, Z622) used at 1 : 400 dilution (3). Fixation: Omnifix II or 4% paraformaldehyde in 0.1 M sodium phosphate, pH 7, either fixative for 10 min at room temperature. Permeablize with 0.1–0.2% Triton X-100 in PBS. Visualize with FITC goat anti-rabbit IgG (Jackson or Kirkegaard-Perry), 1 : 50 dilution.

Acknowledgements

The authors thank Jeff Mumm, Sara Whitehead, and Arthur Lander for their contributions to developing many of the procedures that are referred to in this manuscript. We are grateful to Shelley Plattner and John Busse for photographic work. This work was supported by grants DC02180 and NS32174 from the National Institutes of Health to A. L. Calof.

References

1. Mackay-Sim, A. and Kittel, P. (1991). *J. Neurosci.*, **11,** 979.
2. Graziadei, P. P. C. and Monti Graziadei, G. A. (1978). In *Handbook of sensory physiology, Volume IX: Development of sensory systems* (ed. M. Jacobson), pp. 55–83. Springer-Verlag, New York.
3. Calof, A. L. and Chikaraishi, D. M. (1989). *Neuron*, **3,** 115.
4. Calof, A. L., Lander, A. D., and Chikaraishi, D. M. (1991). In *Regeneration of vertebrate sensory receptor cells* (ed. G. R. Bock and J. Whelan), pp. 249–65. John Wiley and Sons, Chichester.
5. DeHamer, M. K., Guevara, J. L., Hannon, K., Olwin, B. B., and Calof, A. L. (1994). *Neuron*, **13,** 1083.
6. Holcomb, J. D., Mumm, J. S., and Calof, A. L. (1995). *Dev. Biol.*, in press.
7. Calof, A. L. and Lander, A. D. (1991). *J. Cell Biol.*, **115,** 779.
8. Calof, A. L., Campanero, M. R., O'Rear, J. J., Yurchenco, P. D., and Lander, A. D. (1994). *Neuron*, **13,** 117.
9. Farbman, A. I. (1977). *Anat. Rec.*, **189,** 187.
10. Noble, M., Mallaburn, P. S., and Klein, N. (1984). *Neurosci. Lett.*, **45,** 193.

11. Schubert, D., Stallcup, W., LaCorbiere, M., Kidokoro, Y., and Orgel, L. (1985). *Proc. Natl. Acad. Sci. USA*, **82,** 7782.
12. Gonzales, F., Farbman, A. I., and Gesteland, R. C. (1985). *J. Neurosci. Meth.*, **14,** 77.
13. Chuah, M. I., Farbman, A. I., and Menco, B. P. M. (1985). *Brain Res.*, **338,** 259.
14. Chuah, M. I., David, S., and Blaschuk, O. (1991). *Dev. Brain Res.*, **60,** 123.
15. Coon, H. G., Curcio, F., Sakaguchi, K., Brandi, M. L., and Swerdlow, R. D. (1989). *Proc. Natl. Acad. Sci. USA*, **86,** 1703.
16. Pixley, S. K. and Pun, R. Y. K. (1990). *Dev. Brain Res.*, **53,** 125.
17. Ronnett, G. V., Hester, L. D., and Snyder, S. H. (1991). *J. Neurosci.*, **11,** 1243.
18. Calof, A. L., Adusumalli, M., DeHamer, M. K., Guevara, J. L., Mumm, J., Whitehead, S., *et al.* (1994). In *Olfaction and taste XI* (ed. K. Kurihara, N. Suzuki, and H. Ogawa), pp. 36–40. Springer-Verlag, Tokyo.
19. Danciger, E., Mettline, C., Vidal, M., Morris, R., and Margolis, F. (1989). *Proc. Natl. Acad. Sci. USA*, **86,** 8565.
20. Guillemot, F., Lo, L. C., Johnson, J. E., Auerbach, A., Anderson, D. J., and Joyner, A. L. (1993). *Cell*, **75,** 463.
21. Calof, A. L., Escandon, E., Guevara, J. L., Mumm, J. S., Nikolics, K., and Whitehead, S. J. (1993). *Mol. Biol. Cell*, **4,** 371a.
22. Calof, A. L., Adusumalli, M. D., DeHamer, M., Guevara, J. L., Mumm, J. S., and Whitehead, S. J. (1994). *J. Cell. Biochem.*, **S18B,** 171.
23. Prouty, S. M. and Levitt, P. (1993). *J. Comp. Neurol.*, **332,** 444.
24. Calof, A. L. and Guevara, J. L. (1993). *NeuroProtocols*, **3,** 222.
25. Bottenstein, J. E. and Sato, G. H. (1979). *Proc. Natl. Acad. Sci. USA*, **76,** 514.
26. Gennarini, G., Rougon, G., Deagostini-Bazin, H., Hirn, M., and Goridis, C. (1984). *Eur. J. Biochem.*, **142,** 65.
27. Pixley, S. K. (1992). *Glia*, **5,** 269.
28. Devon, R. and Doucette, R. (1992). *Brain Res.*, **589,** 175.

16

Schwann cell culture

LOUISE MORGAN

1. Introduction

Schwann cells support neuronal function in the intact nerve by supplying the myelin sheath around larger axons. Schwann cells are likely to also regulate the ionic environment of axons, provide neurotrophic support, and regulate the periaxonal space. During development and after nerve injury, Schwann cells provide increased neurotrophic support for neurons both as a source of soluble neurotrophic factors and by providing a growth promoting substrate for axonal regrowth by synthesis of permissive molecules both on the cell surface and secreted into the extracellular matrix (1).

Cultures of Schwann cells facilitate analysis of both normal Schwann cell function and of disease where the primary effect is on Schwann cell function. Diseases in this category include neurofibromatosis, associated with loss of Schwann cell growth control, the hereditary peripheral neuropathy Charcot-Marie-Tooth disease, and the immune-mediated polyneuropathy Guillan Barré syndrome, both of which are demyelinating diseases, and leprosy which is associated with loss of function by both non-myelin and myelin-forming Schwann cells (2).

In vivo, Schwann cells survive the axonal degeneration that follows a cut or crush injury, at least in the medium-term. Likewise in culture Schwann cells can be maintained for long periods with no axonal contact. Schwann cells can be cultured from any peripheral nerve, and the most commonly used in laboratory animals are the major nerves to the limbs; the sciatic nerves and the brachial plexus. Schwann cells can be isolated from tissue taken for biopsy from human adult or from fetal nerves and cultured in a similar way (3,4).

2. Nerve dissociation

The most widely used method of culturing Schwann cells is to dissociate nerves with enzymes to obtain a suspension of cells which are then maintained in culture (5). The dissection of these nerves from neonatal rat is described in *Protocols 1* and *2* and illustrated in *Figures 1* and *2*.

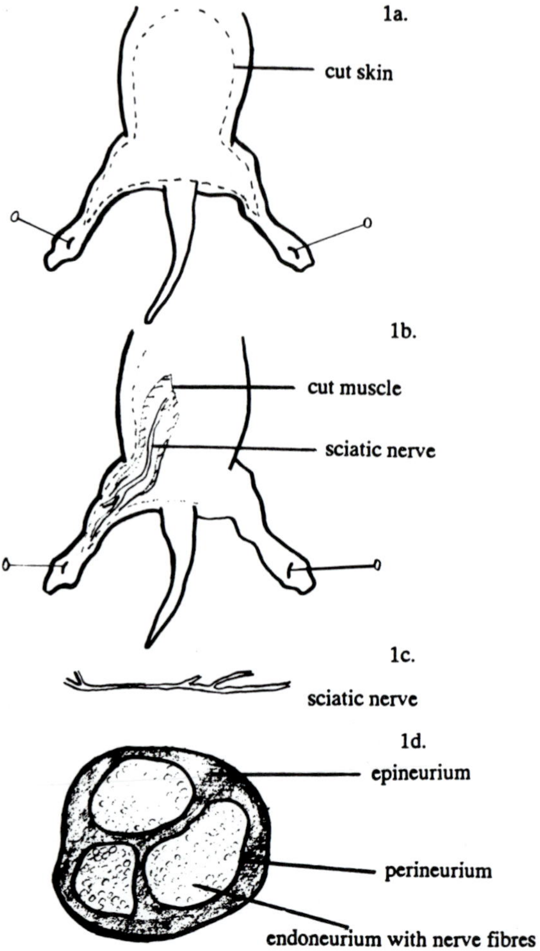

Figure 1. Dissection of neonatal rat sciatic nerve. (a) The animal is killed and pinned out as described in *Protocol 1*. The skin is cut away as shown by the dotted line. (b) The nerve is exposed by carefully cutting away the overlying muscle layers. (c) The nerve is placed in medium for cleaning and desheathing. (d) Transverse section through a peripheral nerve. Several nerve bundles are shown within the epineural sheath. When this is peeled away the endoneurium is still covered by the perineurium.

2.1 Desheathing

The homogeneity of the Schwann cell suspension is enhanced if the epineurium surrounding the nerve is removed (see *Figure 1d*). Most of this connective tissue sheath can be dissected away with forceps. If the nerve has been removed with little damage the epineurium will peel away like removing a stocking.

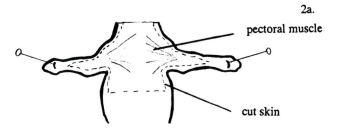

2a.

pectoral muscle

cut skin

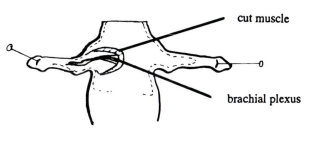

2b.

cut muscle

brachial plexus

2c.

brachial plexus to show interconnecting branches

Figure 2. Dissection of the neonatal rat brachial plexus. (a) The animal is killed and pinned out as described in *Protocol 2*. The skin is cut away as indicated by the dotted line. (b) The pectoral muscle is cut away as indicated. (c) The brachial plexus contains many interconnecting branches, this makes it difficult to clean away the epineural sheath until the branches are cut apart as described in *Protocol 2*.

Protocol 1. Dissection of rat sciatic nerve (*Figure 1*)

Equipment and reagents

- Cork dissecting board covered with aluminium foil and cleaned with 70% ethanol
- Fine tipped and smooth surfaced forceps and fine scissors for handling the dissected nerves, sterilized by immersion in 70% ethanol, dipped in 100% ethanol, and air dried
- Dissecting pins
- Small Petri dish containing Hepes-buffered MEM or L-15 medium on ice
- Coarse scissors and forceps for skin dissection
- A dissecting microscope with fibre-optic lighting is necessary for the desheathing stage of most nerves, and helpful for the main dissection of smaller animals

Method

1. Kill animal by scheduled procedure suitable for age and species.

2. Pin on dissecting board with dorsal side up.

Protocol 1 *Continued*

3. Clean skin with 70% ethanol and cut away as shown (*Figure 1a*).

4. Using scissors cut through the muscle as shown and expose the nerve from where it branches to enter the spinal cord proxomally to below the thigh at the distal end (*Figure 1b*), cutting off the minor branches. The dissection towards the proximal end of the sciatic nerve requires cutting through the pelvic bones, this is not practical for older animals and the nerve should be cut off near the top of the leg.

5. Cut through the ends of the nerve and gently lift it (*Figure 1c*) into cold Hepes-buffered MEM or L-15 medium.

6. Repeat on the other side, pooling the tissue.

7. Clean off any attached fat or muscle tissue and desheath the nerves by holding one end with forceps whilst pulling the epineural sheath away with a second pair of forceps (the layers of the nerve are illustrated in *Figure 1d*). This is easier if the nerve is first cut in half so that the epineural sheath can be pulled away from the centre towards the branches at each end.

8. Dissociate and culture as described in *Protocols 3* or *4*.

Protocol 2. Dissection of rat brachial plexus (*Figure 2*)

Equipment and reagents
- As *Protocol 1*

Method

1. Kill animal as in *Protocol 1*.

2. Pin on dissecting board with ventral side up.

3. Clean skin with 70% ethanol and cut away skin as shown in *Figure 2a*.

4. Using scissors cut through the pectoral muscle to expose the nerves from where they emerge from under the sternum and dissect down the forelimb following the main branches (see *Figure 2b*).

5. Cut through the both ends and gently lift out the bundle of nerves. Place in cold Hepes-buffered MEM or L-15 medium.

6. Repeat on other side, pooling the tissue.

7. Clean off any attached fat or muscle tissue and remove the blood vessels. The plexus is made up of interconnecting strands of nerve as illustrated in *Figure 2c*. Cut the branches of nerve apart so that there are several short, unbranched lengths of nerve and desheath each one as described in *Protocol 1*.

8. Dissociate and culture as described in *Protocols 3* or *4*.

2.2 Dissociation

Protocols 3 and *4* show how to obtain a suspension of Schwann cells from rat nerve tissue. The same methods have been used for human (4) and guinea-pig (6) nerves.

Protocol 3. Dissociation of rat peripheral nerve

This method allows total dissociation of the nerve, but is not suitable if surface antigens to be examined are sensitive to trypsin.

Equipment and reagents

- Ca^{2+}/Mg^{2+}-free solution for enzymes: 84.6 ml double distilled water, 10 ml 10 x Krebs solution, 2 ml 50 x essential amino acids solution, 2.5 ml 7.5% $NaHCO_3$ (sterile), 0.5 ml 0.3% phenol red (sterile), 0.4 ml 50% glucose—warm glucose to dissolve and filter to sterilize
- 10 x Krebs (without Ca^{2+}/Mg^{2+}): 14 g NaCl, 0.7 g KCl, 0.325 g KH_2PO_4,—make up to 200 ml with double distilled water, autoclave to sterilize
- Trypsin-containing enzyme mixture: 2 mg/ml collagenase (Lorne Laboratories Ltd., Twyford, Reading, Berkshire), 1.25 mg/ml trypsin (trypsin 1 : 300, Life Technologies)—dissolve collagenase and trypsin together in Ca^{2+}/Mg^{2+}-free Krebs solution with added essential amino acids, sterilize by filtration

- Dulbecco's modified Eagles medium (DMEM) (if cells are to be kept in an incubator gassed with 5% CO_2, note that commercial DMEM is prepared for 10% CO_2 and will be too alkaline): make up from a 10 x concentrated DMEM preparation, adding 2.5 ml of 7.5% sodium bicarbonate solution for each 100 ml—add 100 U/ml each of penicillin and streptomycin, 5 µg/ml insulin, 1 mM glutamine, and 10% calf serum
- Laminin treated tissue culture substrates: coat poly-L-lysine treated plastic for 1 h at room temperature with laminin 10 µg/ml in DMEM (Sigma), do not attempt to bring to pH 7.4 with CO_2 as laminin binds better at alkaline pH; remove laminin solution immediately before adding cells, do not dry (laminin is used at 20 µg/ml on poly-L-lysine coated glass coverslips)

Method

1. Dissect nerves as *Protocols 1, 2,* or *6*.

2. Place nerves in enzyme in a fresh Petri dish, cut small (about 1 mm) and incubate in 37 °C incubator containing 5% CO_2 and 95% air for the times indicated below. Gently shake the tissue at 30 min intervals and add an equal volume of fresh enzyme after 30 min and again after 1 h.

   Time in enzymes:

embryo–10 days	40 min
10 days–15 days	1 h
15 days–adult	3 x 30 min

   Use 500 µl of enzymes for the sciatic nerves and brachial plexus dissected from one neonatal rat, and 500 µl for each 1 cm of adult nerve.

3. At the end of the incubation add an equal volume of calf serum and gently triturate the tissue (take the tissue slowly up and down in a plastic tip attached to an automatic pipette).

Protocol 3. *Continued*

4. Spin the resulting cell suspension at 500 *g* for 10 min, remove the supernatant, and resuspend the pellet in culture medium.

5. Count the cells[a] and plate in DMEM with 10% calf serum on laminin coated poly-L-lysine treated tissue culture plastic or glass coverslips.

[a] If the nerve is well myelinated it will be impossible to count the cells at this stage.

Protocol 4. Dissociation of rat peripheral nerve in trypsin-free enzymes

This method preserves trypsin-sensitive surface proteins and is especially suitable for fragile tissue, for example embryonic nerves.

Equipment and reagents

● Trypsin-free enzyme cocktail: 2 mg/ml collagenase (Lorne Laboratories Ltd.), 1.2 mg/ml hyaluronidase (Sigma), 0.3 mg/ml trypsin inhibitor from chicken egg white (Sigma)—dissolve the enzymes in Ca^{2+}/Mg^{2+}-free Krebs with added essential amino acids (see *Protocol 3*), filter to sterilize

Method

1. Proceed as *Protocol 3*, steps 1–5, using the times and volumes indicated below.

2. Times in enzyme cocktail:

   embryo   1 h
   0–10 days   1.25 h
   10 days–adult   2.75 h: add an equal volume of fresh enzyme at 1 h.

3. Use 500 μl to dissociate the sciatic nerves from eight embryonic rats, 500 μl for the sciatic nerves and brachial plexus from each one- to ten-day-old rat, and 500 μl for each 1 cm of adult sciatic nerve.

2.3 Schwann cell yield

Using *Protocol 3*, and after treatment with cytosine arabinoside to deplete the fibroblast population (see below), 7–8 x 10^5 Schwann cells are obtained from one six-day-old rat when the Schwann cells from the sciatic nerves and brachial plexus are pooled, and, of this approximately 66% are from the sciatic nerve and 33% from the brachial plexus. The same methods will yield approximately 10000 cells from the (unmyelinated) cervical sympathetic nerve trunks of one six-day-old rat or approximately 30000 cells/cm of nerve from adult rat cervical sympathetic nerve trunk, see *Protocol 6* for this dissection. Adult rat sciatic nerve yields only about 600 cells/mg of tissue (7).

3. Maintaining Schwann cells *in vitro*

Schwann cells can be maintained in DMEM with added serum, insulin, glutamine, and antibiotics (see *Protocol 3*, Equipment and reagents). Schwann cells will attach to poly-L-lysine treated tissue culture plastic; however, attachment is often enhanced if the surface is laminin coated. Freshly isolated Schwann cells can be plated on poly-L-lysine and laminin treated tissue culture plastic then, after purification, re-plated on to a new substrate. *Protocol 5* describes how to passage Schwann cells. One advantage of passaging the cells is that only after the myelin-forming cells have de-differentiated (after about four days in culture) can an accurate estimate of cell numbers be made.

Protocol 5.   Secondary Schwann cells

Equipment and reagents

- PBS/EDTA: 1 litre PBS (Ca^{2+}/Mg^{2+}-free) with 5×10^{-4} M EDTA and 5 ml of 0.3% phenol red (add NaOH to dissolve phenol red stock solution), autoclave
- Trypsin: 0.125 mg/ml trypsin (trypsin 1 : 300, Life Technologies) dissolved in PBS/EDTA, sterilized by filtration

Method

1. Remove medium and wash cells in PBS/EDTA.

2. Remove PBS/EDTA and add more PBS/EDTA containing 0.125 mg/ml trypsin.[a]

3. Warm to 37 °C until cells detach from the culture substrate.

4. Add serum to inhibit the trypsin and centrifuge cells at 500 *g* for 10 min.

5. Resuspend the cells in fresh culture medium, count, and re-plate.

6. Secondary Schwann cells are often difficult to plate on poly-L-lysine plastic or glass coverslips, attachment is improved if the substrate is laminin treated (see *Protocol 3*).

[a] It is possible to remove the cells without trypsin; if trypsin is left out at this stage the cells will detach from the dish if they are left longer at 37 °C.

3.1 Schwann cell purification

Desheathed nerve contains cells from the perineurium, endoneurial fibroblasts and macrophages, and cells from blood vessels, in addition to Schwann cells. The majority of the contaminating cells that survive in culture have fibroblast-like morphology. Cultures from six-day-old rat peripheral nerve contain only about 6% fibroblastic cells after 24 hours. However, Schwann cells proliferate slowly in most culture media, and with time the faster dividing fibroblasts become the predominant cell. Various strategies can be used to remove the fibroblasts, some of these are given here.

(a) Treatment with antimitotic drugs. This method takes advantage of the fact that Schwann cells divide slowly in culture medium containing 10% serum, whilst serum is a potent mitogen for fibroblasts. The cytotoxic drug cytosine arabinoside (10^{-5} M) can be added to Schwann cells in 10% calf serum after 24 h in culture and left for 72 h before washing. If the serum concentration is now reduced to 1% the few remaining fibroblasts will proliferate slowly and not take over the culture.

Cytosine arabinoside is generally sufficient to reduce the fibroblastic cell contamination to an acceptable level, especially if nerves have been desheathed before dissociation. However, in the mouse, serum is a mitogen for Schwann cells. In this case cytosine arabinoside will also kill Schwann cells and in these cultures Schwann cell purification will require a different strategy. A similar problem is encountered when Schwann cells are taken from embryonic rat sciatic nerve; these cells die if they are treated with cytosine arabinoside. As there is a high rate of Schwann cell DNA synthesis in the nerve at this stage of development (8) this death may be due to antimitotic effects of cytosine arabinoside. However as the cells are plated in medium that is not mitogenic for postnatal Schwann cells, and as cytosine arabinoside is not added until after 24 h in culture it is unlikely that these cells are dividing. This raises the possibility that cytosine arabinoside is toxic for embryonic Schwann cells in the absence of DNA synthesis, as it is for postmitotic chick embryonic sensory and parasympathetic neurons (9).

(b) Immunolabelling and complement killing. Rat fibroblasts differ from Schwann cells in expressing Thy-1.1 on the cell surface. After dissociation or after four days culture cells can be incubated with antibody to Thy-1.1 and rabbit complement to kill fibroblastic cells without affecting the Schwann cells (5). It is necessary to screen batches of complement that are not toxic for Schwann cells. However, as not all fibroblasts express Thy-1.1, there will be residual contamination when this method is used.

(c) Differential adhesion. Fibroblasts attach to poly-L-lysine coated glass more readily than Schwann cells. Kreider and co-workers (10) take advantage of this difference to selectively remove fibroblasts from cell suspensions dissociated from neonatal rat sciatic nerves.

(d) Differential trypsinization. Using 1.25 mg/ml trypsin for 20 sec on cultured mouse Schwann cells it is possible to selectively remove Schwann cells from the tissue culture plate surface leaving most of the fibroblasts behind (11). A similar enrichment for Schwann cells is seen in cultures of adult rat sciatic nerve where 0.25 mg/ml trypsin in PBS/EDTA at 37 °C for 2–3 min will selectively remove Schwann cells. This reduces the fibroblast contamination, but greatly decreases the the final Schwann cell yield (Dr Z. Dong, personal communication).

(e) Panning with antibodies. Antibodies attached to tissue culture plastic can be used to selectively remove a subpopulation of cells from a mixed suspension. Positive or negative selection is possible (see Chapter 8). Battacharyya and co-workers (12) used the monoclonal antibody to the myelin protein P_o 1E8 to positively select for Schwann cells from dissociated embryonic chick sciatic nerve.

(f) Serum starvation. Fibroblasts do not divide in serum-free medium. Dubois-Dalcq and co-workers (13) were able to maintain mouse Schwann cells *in vitro* entirely without serum and the cultures were not overgrown by fibroblasts. The phenotype of these cells, however, is not the same as similar cells maintained in serum since they do not fully de-differentiate and it takes more than two weeks to remove myelin debris.

4. Alternative methods for culturing Schwann cells

The methods described in *Protocols 3* and *4* will liberate Schwann cells from any nerve. They are most suitable for unmyelinated nerves or for nerves taken before myelination is complete, and the yield will be reduced where there is a high per cent of myelinated axons. This is not because these cells are killed by the enzyme treatment and subsequent trituration, but rather due to a failure of the very large myelin-forming cells to attach to the culture substrate. Myelin-forming cells tend to form a floating raft of tissue, and only a few attach to the substrate. It is possible to maximize the number of myelin-forming cells by carefully reducing the plating density until the cells do not attach to each other, however, where large numbers of cells are required one of the following methods may be more suitable. The disadvantage of the methods described below is the delay between the cells losing axonal contact and obtaining a culture of pure Schwann cells.

(a) Nerve explants. Morrissey and co-workers (14) maintained explants of nerve from adult rat and human in culture. Schwann cells divide in the explant in a similar way to that seen during Wallerian degeneration *in vivo*. The explants are cut out of the culture and moved to a new dish every seven to ten days and cells migrate out of the explant on to the culture substrate. During the first passages the cells migrating out are a mixture of Schwann cells and fibroblasts, however after several moves the cells migrating on to the culture substrate are almost entirely Schwann cells. After four to five weeks the explant is dissociated to give cultures greatly enriched for Schwann cells.

(b) Nerve explants with mitogens. Rutkowski and co-workers (3) maintained explants of adult human sural nerve in culture for up to 14 days in

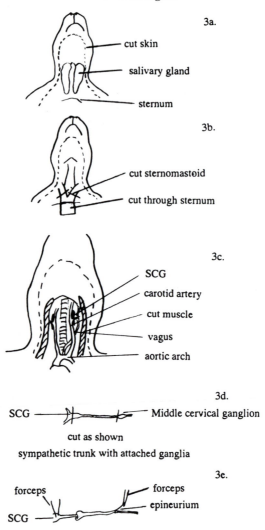

3a.

— cut skin

— salivary gland

— sternum

3b.

— cut sternomastoid

— cut through sternum

3c.

SCG

carotid artery

— cut muscle

— vagus

— aortic arch

3d.

SCG ——— Middle cervical ganglion

cut as shown

sympathetic trunk with attached ganglia

3e.

forceps — forceps

— epineurium

SCG —

Desheathing the sympathetic trunk

Figure 3. Dissection of the neonatal rat sympathetic trunk. (a) The animal is killed as described in *Protocol 6* and pinned out as shown. The skin is cut away as indicated by the dotted line to expose the salivary glands underneath. (b) The salivary glands are removed and the underlying muscles and the anterior part of the sternum cut away or deflected until the trachea, carotid arteries, and aortic arch can be seen. (c) The SCG is located under the first major branch from the carotid artery. (d) The SCG with attached sympathetic trunk are dissected free from the surrounding tissues and cut as shown. (e) The trunk can be desheathed in a similar way to larger mixed nerves, but due to the small size of the nerve this procedure takes practice.

medium containing Schwann cell mitogens and then dissociated the tissue. This gave a 25-fold increase in yield compared to cultures where cells were dissociated from the nerve immediately.

(c) Schwann cells dissociated from cut or crushed nerve. During Wallerian degeneration after axons are severed there is considerable Schwann cell proliferation. If cut nerves are allowed to degenerate and then dissociated as described in *Protocols 3* or *4* the Schwann cell yield will be greatly increased. This is first due to the presence of more Schwann cells in the nerve, secondly to greater attachment to the culture substrate due to enhanced expression of adhesion molecules, and thirdly to the cells containing less myelin (15,16). It should be noted that at early stages of development in the rat prior denervation will not increase the Schwann cell yield (17).

(d) Myelin-forming and non-myelin Schwann cells. *In vivo* Schwann cells are not all the same, since only those in association with large axons synthesize a myelin sheath. Most nerves are mixed, containing some axons with a diameter above and others below the threshold for myelination. There are, however, some nerves with mostly small (cervical sympathetic trunk nerve in the rat) or mostly large (ventral root) axons. Schwann cells taken from these nerves will be enriched for non-myelin Schwann cells, or myelin-forming Schwann cells respectively. *Figure 3* and *Protocol 6* illustrate the dissection of neonatal rat cervical sympathetic trunk. Cultures of cervical sympathetic trunk contain only 0.5% myelin-forming Schwann cells. However these cultures will contain a few sympathetic neurons (18).

Protocol 6.   Dissection of rat cervical sympathetic trunk (*Figure 3*)

Equipment and reagents

• As *Protocol 1*, but a dissecting microscope with fibre-optic lighting is essential for this dissection

Method

1. Kill by overdose of anaesthetic and bleed out by cutting through the heart.

2. Pin on dissecting board with ventral side up.

3. Clean skin with 70% ethanol and cut away as shown in *Figure 3a*.

4. Remove the salivary gland, cut through the sternomastoid muscles, and cut out the central bone of the sternum as shown in *Figure 3b*.

5. Remove the thymus gland to expose the aortic arch and cut out or deflect the sternohyoid muscles as shown in *Figure 3c*. Locate the carotid artery and follow it forwards to the first branch. Locate the

---

Protocol 6 *Continued*

pale superior cervical ganglion (SCG) under the fork in the artery (see *Figure 3c*). Do not confuse with the nearby nodose ganglion on the vagus nerve; this is shiny white due to the presence of myelin whilst the unmyelinated SCG is translucent making it easy to differentiate between the two.

6. Cut out in a bundle the artery, SCG, and vagus nerve down to the aortic arch. Place the tissue in cold Hepes-buffered MEM or L-15 medium. Gently dissect the SCG away from the surounding tissue. The cervical sympathetic trunk connects the SCG with the middle cervical ganglion located beside the aortic arch and is embedded in connective tissue beside the blood vessels and the larger vagus nerve. Gently tease the fragile cervical sympathetic trunk free keeping the SCG attached.

7. If the smaller middle cervical ganglion is attached, remove this and cut the SCG in half before deheathing as shown in *Figures 3c* and *3d*. Cut off the remaining piece of SCG before dissociating as described in *Protocols 3* or *4*.

(e) Co-cultures of Schwann cells and neurons. Schwann cells do not maintain their mature phenotype when they are kept in culture. When Schwann cells are co-cultured with neurons, however, they will interact with the neurites and can synthesize a myelin sheath *in vitro*, provided they are given vitamin C, a necessary constituent for collagen synthesis, and serum. Myelin synthesis can be co-ordinated *in vitro* by withholding vitamin C until all the Schwann cells associating with larger neurites are in a pre-myelin state then, when vitamin C is added, myelination will follow (19). Mature non-myelin forming Schwann cells co-cultured with sympathetic neurons have also been described (20).

5. Manipulation of Schwann cells *in vitro*

5.1 Schwann cell mitogens

Table 1 lists Schwann cell mitogens. cAMP elevation is necessary as a co-mitogen for most Schwann cell growth factors, however TGFb can partially replace cAMP elevation, acting as a co-mitogen with PDGF, aFGF, and bFGF for rat Schwann cells (26).

5.2 Use of mitogens to expand Schwann cell numbers

It is possible to obtain large numbers of Schwann cells using mitogens *in vitro*. The doubling time of Schwann cells cultured in the presence of glial growth factor and the reversible activator of adenylate cyclase, forskolin, is two days (35). Therefore, starting with 5×10^5 cells taken from one neonatal

Table 1. Rat Schwann cell mitogens

	Activity			
	No serum		**Serum**	
cAMP elevating drugs	–	+	–	+
Treatment				
Defined medium	–	–	–	+ (21,22)
Plasma	–	±	nd	nd (21)
GGF*#	–	++	+	++ (21,23,24)
TGFβ–1	±	±	+	++ (21,25,26)
TGFβ–2	nd	nd	+	++ (21)
FGF–1	nd	nd	±	++ (27)
FGF–2	–	++	±	++ (21,24,26,27)
PDGF–AB	–	++	±	++ (21,24,27,28)
PDGF–BB	–	++	±	++ (21,28)
NDGF#	+	nd	nd	nd (29)
Axon contact#	+	nd	+	nd (30)
Axon enriched fragments#	+	nd	+	nd (31,32)
Myelin enriched fragments#	nd	nd	+	nd (32)
Neuron–derived pa urokinase#	+	++	nd	nd (33)

Key:
+, active as mitogen; ++, enhanced activity with cAMP elevation; –, not mitogenic; ±, reports vary.
GGF, glial growth factor. *This factor has recently been demonstrated to be identical to the neu differentiation factor heregulin and aria, a muscle differentiation inducing factor isolated from brain (34).
TGFβ, transforming growth factor β (R&D Systems, Abingdon, Oxon, UK). FGF, fibroblast growth factor (R&D Systems, Abingdon, Oxon, UK). PDGF, platelet-derived growth factor (R&D Systems, Abingdon, Oxon, UK). NDGF, neuron-derived growth factor. pa, plasminogen activator.
nd, not determined. #, not commercially available.
References are given in brackets.

rat it is possible to obtain 8 x 10^6 cells within eight days, providing the cells are not allowed to reach confluence and so inhibit their own division. Porter and co-workers (36) used forskolin and semipure glial growth factor to expand Schwann cell numbers over several months. For the first four months the cells showed no detectable differences from primary Schwann cell cultures in respect to phenotype, basal division rates, and the ability to form myelin on contact with axons when the mitogens were removed. After four months, however, the cells became mitogen-independent, and after 16 months (56 passages) the cells lost the ability to form myelin and formed tumours *in vivo* (37). A similar transformation is seen when Schwann cells are maintained in culture for long times in serum-containing medium with no added growth factors (38,39). The use of expanded or long-term cultured Schwann cells should be treated with caution as the point at which the cells begin to transform has not been closely defined. This is obviously most important if the cells are to be used in experiments where implanted Schwann cells are used to improve nerve regeneration.

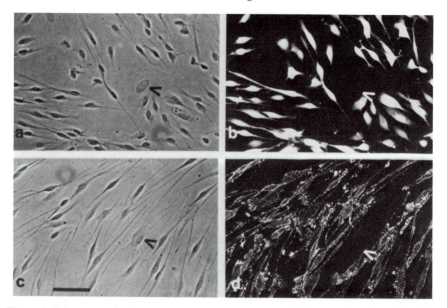

Figure 4. Schwann cells in culture. Neonatal rat Schwann cells in primary culture after enriching for Schwann cells by treatment with cytosine arabinoside. (a) Schwann cells with typical bipolar morphology, phase-contrast. (b) S100 label of the same field of cells, epifluoresence. The flatter cell indicated can be identified as a contaminating cell as it does not express the protein S100, a marker commonly used to distinguish Schwann cells from fibroblasts. (c) Schwann cells, phase-contrast. (d) Low affinity NGF receptor (p75) antibody label of the same field of cells, epifluoresence. The Schwann cells are identified by binding of the antibody to the low affinity NGF receptor, whilst the contaminating cell (indicated) does not express this antigen. Scale bar 58 μm.

6. Schwann cell phenotype *in vitro*

Figure 4 illustrates the typical bipolar morphology of Schwann cells in culture. Contaminating cells are flat cells that do not express the Schwann cell markers S100 or the low affinity NGF receptor p75. Schwann cells change with time in culture, Schwann cell phenotype in culture and in the intact nerve is described in full in a review by Mirsky and Jessen (40).

Differentiation of Schwann cells *in vitro* towards the myelin-forming phenotype can be induced by drugs that elevate cAMP, provided that growth factors that act as a co-mitogen with elevated cAMP are not present (41).

7. Schwann cells from various species

Table 2 shows some of the many species from which Schwann cells have been cultured. Different species vary in the time course of development, for example guinea-pig sciatic nerve is well myelinated at birth, whilst in the neonatal

Table 2. Schwann cells maintained *in vitro* from various species

Species	Embryonic	Neonatal	Adult
Rat	42	5	14,7
Mouse	–	11	16
Cat	–	–	43
Human	4	–	3
Rabbit	–	44	44
Guinea-pig	–	6	–
Pig	–	45	–
Chick	12	–	–
Quail	46	46	46

Numbers indicate reference number.

Table 3. Schwann cell lines and genetically manipulated Schwann cells

Cell line	Species	How made	Can form myelin
218	nn-rat-sn	SpTr-cult	nd (38)
1.17	nn-rat-sn	SpTr-cult	Yes (36)
iSC	ad-rat	SpTr-cult	nd (16)
RN-22	Rat	ENU	nd (48)
D6P2T	Rat	ENU	nd (49)
33B	Rat	ENU	nd (50)
JS1 schwannoma	Rat CNS	ENU-pn-inj	nd (51)
1° schwannoma	Rat	ENU	nd (52)
MSC 80	nn-mouse	SpTr-cult	Yes (39)
1° NF-1 cells	Human		nd (53)
1° schwannoma	Human		nd (54)

Schwann cells genetically modified in culture

–	nn-rat-sn		No (55)
MT₄H1	nn-rat-sn		nd (56)
LT5	nn-rat-sn		nd (57)
–	nn-rat-sn		Yes (58)
MS1	ad-mouse-DRG + nerve		nd (59)

Key:
ENU, transplacental induction after intraperitoneal ethylnitrosourea injection of pregnant female.
ENU-pn-inj, postnatal injection of ethylnitrosourea.
SpTr-cult, spontaneous transformation in culture.
nn, neonatal; sn, sciatic nerve; DRG, dorsal root ganglion; nd, not determined.
References are given in brackets.

rat sciatic nerve the first myelin sheaths are only just beginning to form. Schwann cells from all species de-differentiate in culture although the extent and time course of this de-differentiation varies between species (47). One other important difference between species is in the response to mitogens, for example, serum is a mitogen for mouse but not rat Schwann cells (11,21) and mitogens for adult human Schwann cells have not yet been defined.

8. Transformed Schwann cells and schwannoma cell lines

Table 3 lists Schwann cell and schwannoma lines and cell lines derived by transformation of Schwann cells *in vitro* by the insertion of oncogenes.

References

1. Fawcett, J. W. and Keynes, R. J. (1990). *Annu. Rev. Neurosci.*, **13,** 43.
2. Dyck, P. J., Thomas, P. K., Lambert, E. H., and Bunge, R. (1984). *Peripheral neuropathy.* W. B. Saunders Company.
3. Rutkowski, J. L., Tennekoon, G. I., and McGullicuddy, J. E. (1992). *Ann. Neurol.*, **31,** 580.
4. Samuel, N. M., Mirsky, R., Grange, J. M., and Jessen, K. R. (1987). *Clin. Exp. Immunol.*, **68,** 500.
5. Brockes, J. P., Fields, K. L., and Raff, M. C. (1979). *Brain Res.*, **165,** 105.
6. Eccleston, P. A., Jessen, K. R., and Mirsky, R. (1987). *Dev. Biol.*, **124,** 409.
7. Scarpini, E., Kreider, B. Q., Lisak, R. P., and Pleasure, D. E. (1988). *Exp. Neurol.*, **102,** 167.
8. Stewart, H. J. S., Morgan, L., Jessen, K. R., and Mirsky, R. (1993). *Eur. J. Neurosci.*, **5,** 1136.
9. Wallace, T. L. and Johnson, E. M. (1989). *J. Neurosci.*, **9,** 115.
10. Kreider, B. Q., Messing, A., Doan, H., Kim, S. U., Lisak, R. P., and Pleasure, D. (1981). *Brain Res.*, **207,** 433.
11. White, F. V., Ceccarini, C., Georgieff, I., Matthieu, J.-M., and Costantino-Ceccarini, E. (1983). *Exp. Cell Res.*, **148,** 183.
12. Bhattacharyya, A., Brackenbury, R., and Ratner, N. (1993). *J. Neurosci. Res.*, **35,** 1.
13. Dubois-Dalcq, M., Rentier, B., Baron, A., van Evercooren, N., and Burge, B. W. (1981). *Exp. Cell Res.*, **131,** 283.
14. Morrissey, T. K., Kleitman, N., and Bunge, R. P. (1991). *J. Neurosci.*, **11,** 2433.
15. Komiyama, A., Novicki, D. L., and Suzuki, K. (1991). *J. Neurosci. Res.*, **29,** 308.
16. Bolin, L. M., Isimaa, T. P., and Shooter, E. M. (1992). *J. Neurosci. Res.*, **33,** 231.
17. Komiyama, A. and Suzuki, K. (1992). *Brain Res.*, **573,** 267.
18. Jessen, K. R., Morgan, L., Brammer, M., and Mirsky, R. (1985). *J. Cell Biol.*, **101,** 1135.
19. Eldridge, C. F., Bunge, M. B., Bunge, R. P., and Wood, P. M. (1987). *J. Cell Biol.*, **105,** 1023.
20. Obremski, V. J., Johnson, M. I., and Bunge, M. B. (1993). *J. Neurocytol.*, **22,** 102.
21. Davis, J. B. and Stroobant, P. (1990). *J. Cell Biol.*, **110,** 1353.
22. Raff, M. C., Hornby-Smith, A., and Brockes, J. P. (1978). *Nature*, **273,** 672.
23. Brockes, J. P., Fryxel, K. J., and Lemke, G. E. (1981). *J. Exp. Biol.*, **95,** 215.
24. Stewart, H. J. S., Eccleston, P. A., Jessen, K. R., and Mirsky, R. (1991). *J. Neurosci. Res.*, **30,** 346.
25. Eccleston, P. A., Jessen, K. R., and Mirsky, R. (1989). *J. Neurosci. Res.*, **24,** 524.
26. Schubert, D. (1992). *J. Neurobiol.*, **23,** 143.
27. Chen, J.-K., Yau, L.-L., and Jenq, C.-B. (1991). *J. Neurosci. Res.*, **30,** 321.

28. Eccleston, P. A., Collarini, E. J., Jessen, K. R., Mirsky, R., and Richardson, W. D. (1990). *Eur. J. Neurosci.*, **2**, 985.

29. Nordlund, M., Hong, D., Fei, X., and Ratner, N. (1992). *Glia*, **5**, 182.

30. Moya, F., Bunge, M. B., and Bunge, R. P. (1980). *Proc. Natl. Acad. Sci. USA*, **77**, 6902.

31. Sobue, G., Kreider, B., Asbury, A., and Pleasure, D. (1983). *Brain Res.*, **280**, 263.

32. Yoshino, J., Dinneen, M. P., Lewis, B. L., Meador-Woodruff, J. H, and DeVries, G. H. (1984). *J. Cell Biol.*, **99**, 2303.

33. Baron-Van Evercooren, A., Leprince, P., Rogister, B., Lefebvre, P. P., Delree, P., Selak, I., *et al.* (1987). *Dev. Brain Res.*, **36**, 101.

34. Marchionni, M. A., Goodearl, A. D. J., Chen, M. S., Bermingham-McDonogh, O., Kirk, C., Hendricks, M. *et al.* (1993). *Nature*, **362**, 312.

35. Porter, S., Clarke, M. B., Glazer, L., and Bunge, R. P. (1986). *J. Neurosci.*, **6**, 3070.

36. Porter, S., Glaser, L., and Bunge, R. P. (1987). *Proc. Natl. Acad. Sci. USA*, **84**, 7768.

37. Langford, L. A., Porter, S., and Bunge, R. P. (1988). *J. Neurocytol.*, **17**, 521.

38. Eccleston, P. A., Mirsky, R., and Jessen, K. R. (1991). *Development*, **112**, 33.

39. Boutry, J.-M., Hauw, J.-J., Gransmüller, A., Di-Bert, N., Pouchelet, M., and Baron-Van Evercooren, A. (1992). *J. Neurosci. Res.*, **32**, 15.

40. Mirsky, R. and Jessen, K. R. (1990). *Semin. Neurosci.*, **2**, 423.

41. Morgan, L., Jessen, K. R., and Mirsky, R. (1991). *J. Cell Biol.*, **112**, 457.

42. Mirsky, R., Dubois, C., Morgan, L., and Jessen, K. R. (1990). *Development*, **109**, 105.

43. Wrathall, J. R., Rigamonti, D. D., and Kao, C. C. (1981). *Brain Res.*, **224**, 218.

44. Howe, J. R. and Ritchie, J. M. (1990). *J. Physiol.*, **425**, 169.

45. Kioussi, C. and Matas, R. (1991). *J. Neurochem.*, **57**, 431.

46. Dulac, C., Cameron-Curry, P., Ziller, C., and Le Douarin, N. M. (1988). *Neuron*, **1**, 211.

47. Burrioni, D., White, F. V., Ceccarini, C., Matthieu, J.-M., and Constantino-Ceccarini, E. (1988). *J. Neurochem.*, **50**, 331.

48. Pfeiffer, S. and Wechsler, W. (1972). *Proc. Natl. Acad. Sci. USA*, **69**, 2885.

49. Bansal, R. and Pfeiffer, S. E. (1987). *J. Neurochem.*, **49**, 1902.

50. Fields, K. L., Gosling, C., Megson, M., and Stern, P. L. (1975). *Proc. Natl. Acad. Sci. USA*, **72**, 1286.

51. Kimura, H., Fischer, W. H., and Schubert, D. (1990). *Nature*, **348**, 257.

52. Nikitin, A. Y., Lennartz, K., Pozharisski, K. M., and Rajewsky, M. F. (1991). *Differentiation*, **48**, 33.

53. Sonnenfeld, K. H., Bernd, P., Sobue, G., Lebwohl, M., and Rubenstein, A. E. (1986). *Cancer Res.*, **46**, 1446.

54. Stenman, G., Kindbolm, L.-G., Johansson, M., and Angervall, L. (1991). *Cancer Genet. Cytogenet.*, **57**, 121.

55. Tennekoon, G. H., Yoshino, J., Peden, K. W. C., Bigbee, J., Rutkowski, J. L., Kishimoto, Y., *et al.* (1987). *J. Cell Biol.*, **105**, 2315.

56. Peden, W. C., Charles, C., Sanders, L., and Tennekoon, G. I. (1989). *Exp. Cell Res.*, **185**, 60.

57. Ridley, A. J., Patterson, H. F., Noble, M., and Land, H. (1988). *EMBO J.*, **7**, 1635.

58. Feltri, M. L., Scherer, S. S., Wrabetz, L., Kamholtz, J., and Shy, M. E. (1992). *Proc. Natl. Acad. Sci. USA*, **89**, 8827.

59. Watabe, K., Yamada, M., Kawamura, T., and Kim, S. U. (1990). *J. Neuropathol. Exp. Neurol.*, **5**, 455.

Index

Index

Index